The attack on disease must not be meddlesome; the desire to do something must be guided by sure argument that good will come of it.

Gibson AG (1933) *The Physician's Art*. Clarendon Press, Oxford.

Screening in Disease Prevention

What works?

Walter W Holland

Emeritus Professor
London School of Economics and Political Science
Health and Social Care
London

and

Susie Stewart

Honorary Research Fellow
University of Glasgow
Glasgow

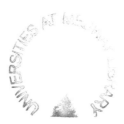

This book is a co-publication between The Nuffield Trust
and the European Observatory on Health Systems and Policies

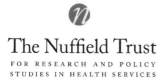

The Nuffield Trust
FOR RESEARCH AND POLICY
STUDIES IN HEALTH SERVICES

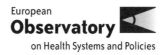

European
Observatory
on Health Systems and Policies

Radcliffe Publishing
Oxford • Seattle

Radcliffe Publishing Ltd
18 Marcham Road
Abingdon
Oxon OX14 1AA
United Kingdom

www.radcliffe-oxford.com
Electronic catalogue and worldwide online ordering facility.

British Library Cataloguing in Publication Data

A catalogue record for this book is available from the British Library.

ISBN 1 85775 770 X

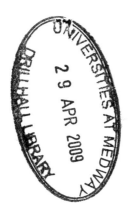

Typeset by Anne Joshua & Associates, Oxford
Printed and bound by TJ International Ltd, Padstow, Cornwall

Contents

About the authors

Walter Holland CBE, FRCP, FFPH qualified from St Thomas's Hospital Medical School in 1954. His entire career has been in medical research. His interests in epidemiology were aroused by his involvement in investigations of the 1957 influenza pandemic while doing his national service in the RAF. After gaining experience at the London School of Hygiene and John Hopkins University School of Hygiene, he returned in 1962 to St Thomas's, where he remained until 1994. His major research interests have been in the epidemiology of chronic respiratory disease, blood pressure and the application of epidemiological principles to health services research. He has published widely, including acting as editor of the *Oxford Textbook of Public Health*. He was President of the International Epidemiological Association and of the Faculty of Public Health Medicine (now the Faculty of Public Health). He has served on many national and international committees concerned with public health, and has spent periods of time in Australia, France, Germany and various parts of the USA. He has had experience of life at the 'sharp end' as a member of a District Management Team, member and vice-chairman of a health authority and non-executive director of a health authority. Susie Stewart and Walter Holland have produced joint publications on several occasions, including *Screening in Health Care* (1990) and *Public Health: the Vision and the Challenge* (1998), both published by the Trust.

Susie Stewart DL, MA, FFPH graduated from St Andrews University in 1962 and obtained a postgraduate diploma in Social Studies from Edinburgh University in 1963. She became an Honorary Member of the Faculty of Public Health Medicine in 1992 and a Fellow in 2001, when she was also appointed an Honorary Research Fellow in the Faculty of Medicine, University of Glasgow. Her career began with a research assistantship in mental handicap and genetic counselling. In 1971 she took up a research and editorial position with Professor Holland in the Department of Community Medicine at St Thomas's Hospital. Following a move back to her home city of Glasgow in 1977, she was for 10 years technical editor of two of the British Medical Association's specialist journals and technical editor for the Panel of Social Medicine and Epidemiology of the Commission of the European Communities. In 1990 she was appointed Executive Secretary of the Scottish Forum for Public Health Medicine and the subsequently established Scottish Needs Assessment Programme. From 1998 to 2000 she acted as Executive Secretary to a Working Group of the Scottish Royal Colleges on Inequalities in Health, and was a member of the Healthy Public Policy Network of the Scottish Council Foundation and editor of the report *The Possible Scot*. She is currently based in the Public Health and Health Policy Section of the Division of Community-Based Sciences at Glasgow University.

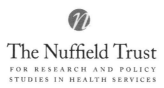

The Nuffield Trust

FOR RESEARCH AND POLICY
STUDIES IN HEALTH SERVICES

The Nuffield Trust is one of the leading independent health policy charitable trusts in the UK. It was established as the Nuffield Provincial Hospitals Trust in 1940 by Viscount Nuffield (William Morris), the founder of Morris Motors. In 1998 the Trustees agreed that the official name of the trust should more fully reflect the Trust's purposes and, in consultation with the Charity Commission, adopted the name The Nuffield Trust for Research and Policy Studies in Health Services, retaining 'The Nuffield Trust' as its working name.

The Nuffield Trust's mission is to promote independent analysis and informed debate on UK healthcare policy. The Nuffield Trust's purpose is to communicate evidence and encourage an exchange around developed or developing knowledge in order to illuminate recognised and emerging issues.

It achieves this through its principal activities:

- bringing together a wide national and international network of people involved in UK healthcare through a series of meetings, workshops and seminars
- commissioning research through its publications and grants programme to inform policy debate
- encouraging inter-disciplinary exchange between clinicians, legislators, academics, healthcare professionals and management, policy makers, industrialists and consumer groups
- supporting evidence-based health policy and practice
- sharing its knowledge in the home countries and internationally through partnerships and alliances.

To find out more, please refer to our website or contact:

The Nuffield Trust
59 New Cavendish St
London
W1G 7LP
Website: www.nuffieldtrust.org.uk
Email: mail@nuffieldtrust.org.uk
Tel: +44 (0)20 7631 8458
Fax: +44 (0)20 7631 8451

Charity number: 209201

List of Trustees

Acknowledgements

We are extremely grateful to the following friends and colleagues who have given us their views on screening and commented on various sections and drafts of the manuscript: Professor M Adler, Professor E Alberman, Ms S Allin, Dr J Austoker, Mr CJ Black, Professor M Bobrow, Dr M Brodin, Dr G Comstock, Dr J Cooper, Dr D Delnoy, Professor C Dezateux, Sir Liam Donaldson, Ms K Dunnell, Dr R Elliott, Dr M Fitzpatrick, Dr P Fox, Dr M Gill, Professor L Gordis, Dr J Muir Gray, Professor M Harrington, Ms C Heidbrink, Dr RC Holland, Dr S Iliffe, Ms N Jemiai, Professor N Kass, Dr N Klazinga, Mr R Klein, Mr J Lawrence, Mr M Lehman, Dr E Lynge, Dr M McCartney, Professor M McKee, Professor T Marteau, Dr J Melia, Professor D Morrell, Dr E Mossialos, Ms D Nicolaou, Mrs J Patnick, Dr A Raffle, Dr LM Reay, Professor M Reid, Dr F Rose, Dr M Rosen, Dr L Salas, Dr F Sassi, Professor F Schelp, Dr N Segnan, Dr D Snashall, Dr H Stoate MP, Professor D Stone, Dr A Streetly, Professor N Wald, Dr JMG Wilson and Dr WN Wykes.

The opinions we express in this book are, of course, entirely our own and we take full responsibility for them.

Walter Holland
Susie Stewart
June 2005

Chapter 1

Historical background, current definitions and criteria

> Complete freedom from disease is almost incompatible with the process of living.*

Introduction

The practice of screening in healthcare – that is, actively seeking to identify a disease or pre-disease condition in people who are presumed and presume themselves to be healthy – is one that grew rapidly during the twentieth century and now has wide acceptance in our society. In looking back over the years since our previous book on screening was published,[1] it is perhaps surprising how little appears to have changed in the provision of screening services or in the knowledge base of screening in the UK. Organisation and audit of existing programmes have undoubtedly improved and, importantly, there is now a UK National Screening Committee which acts as a central reference point for screening throughout the country. With the exception of genetic screening, where the possibilities have multiplied exponentially – although, as we shall show, there are major ethical and implementation issues in this area – we still have broadly the same programmes and services. What has changed, however, is the public perception and expectations of screening, the focus of media attention on health in general and screening in particular, and an increasing recognition, especially among health professionals, that screening can be harmful as well as helpful.

In this chapter we shall look at the historical background to screening, including the establishment of the National Screening Committee, restate acceptable definitions of the process, revisit the criteria that must be fulfilled before screening is introduced and consider briefly some political issues and public perceptions.

Historical background

The benefits of screening were first demonstrated by the use of mass miniature radiography (MMR) for the identification of individuals with tuberculosis. With the introduction of effective treatment for this condition after the end of the Second World War, the use of MMR became widespread in many western countries, particularly the USA and the UK.

In the late 1950s and early 1960s, special campaigns of mass radiography were used to good effect in Scotland – first in Glasgow and then throughout the country – to try and find the unknown and infectious sufferers from tuberculosis.[2] Andrew Semple, Medical Officer of Health in Liverpool from 1953 to 1974,

---

* Dubos R (1960) *Mirage of Health*. George Allen and Unwin, London.

set up a very successful MMR campaign in that city during which more than 80% of the adult population were screened. In 1953 he had noted that tuberculosis remained an intractable problem, with Liverpool having the highest rates in the country apart from Glasgow. By 1960, Semple was able to report a large reduction in cases, resulting from the campaign, and by 1966 it was possible to close the Central Chest Clinic.[3]

Other Medical Officers of Health, such as Robert Parry and Robert Wofinden with the William Budd Centre in Bristol, had developed the imaginative new concept of the health centre.[4] These centres were intended to provide 'lifetime' preventive care and to develop screening services. Integrated care and screening for pregnant women from the antenatal period through birth in hospital or at home to care in the postnatal period were beginning in a few places, as were more co-ordinated care and surveillance for the elderly, the chronic sick and the mentally ill.

With the reduction in the burden of tuberculosis, the concept of screening began to be considered equally applicable to the control of other chronic diseases. This was shown in particular in the USA, where a law on the control of chronic diseases was passed in the late 1950s. A major review of screening in chronic disease was published in the *Journal of Chronic Disease* in 1955.[5] One of the review's editors, Lester Breslow – Head of the Division of Chronic Disease in the California State Health Department at the time – was a keen advocate of screening in this context. The Commission on Chronic Illness was founded in 1957 and started to publish copiously.[6]

In 1961, Thorner and Remein of the United States Public Health Service published the first comprehensive review of the principles of screening. Its evaluation still remains relevant.[7]

The initial push for screening was particularly evident in North America. One of the first examples of this was the enthusiastic introduction of screening for cancer of the cervix in British Columbia and California. This was reviewed critically by Ahluwalia and Doll,[8] who did not consider that screening was justified on the basis of this experience.

One of the most ardent advocates of screening at this time was Morris Collen, Medical Director of the Kaiser Permanente Health Maintenance Organisation, who was interviewed 20 years later in connection with a history of the programme.[9]

Collen considered that regular screening of adults for a variety of conditions could reduce the costs and utilisation of medical services. As a result, regular screening – or preventive medical examination as it was described – was introduced as a component of subscribing to the Kaiser Permanente HMO, despite the inability to demonstrate clear benefits.

In the UK, possibly because of fewer financial resources for health, screening lagged behind. However, Sir George Godber, the Chief Medical Officer from 1960 to 1973, quickly recognised that screening was an important possible method of delivering preventive healthcare.[10] He therefore despatched Dr JMG Wilson, a senior medical officer in the Ministry of Health, to North America to review and learn about the possibilities and problems. Wilson developed his views and these were later written up with Jungner, a Swedish biochemist, and published as a World Health Organization monograph. This remains a landmark contribution to the field of screening.[11]

The 'women's movement' was also growing at this time, with a particular focus on women's health. As a result of the North American experience and the hope that cervical cytology could prevent cancer of the cervix, demand for a national screening programme began to make itself felt. With the development of family planning and women's health services, cervical smears began to be taken increasingly. The ease of performing these smears meant that they were very popular, and there was little concern at this stage about the effectiveness of the procedure or the need for it. Pathology services, particularly cytology, became overwhelmed with the large number of smears needing examination. At that time, most specimen reporting was carried out by medically qualified pathologists. As a result, other aspects of pathology work, such as post-mortems, were neglected. It has been suggested that the demand for cervical cytology in the 1960s was responsible for the great diminution in the number of post-mortem investigations, which had hitherto been more or less routine.

Stimulated by Wilson, the Ministry of Health and various other groups began to consider the implications of screening as a part of healthcare. The Nuffield Provincial Hospitals Trust, for example, convened a Working Party under the chairmanship of Professor T McKeown, which published its findings in 1968.[12]

That group reached two main conclusions. First, evaluation of ten screening procedures showed that, in six of these, evidence was severely deficient with regard to one or more of the following elements: the natural history of the disease; methods of diagnosis and treatment; operational problems; assessment of benefits and costs.

Secondly, examination of screening procedures in Britain suggested that the existing research and administrative framework for screening should be strengthened. Developments appeared to be needed in three main areas:

1 sharper definition of the requirements of screening and of the state of evidence concerning current programmes
2 promotion of those types of research (large-scale, prolonged, applied and economic) that were not readily accommodated within the present framework
3 meticulous attention to the introduction and development of screening programmes to ensure that they were reliable and co-ordinated within the whole range of health services.

Screening was now at the forefront of the health agenda.

That same year the Ministry of Health had created a Joint Standing Sub-Committee on Screening in Medical Care with the remit of reviewing the evidence for any screening programme and making recommendations on what needed to be done before a programme could be introduced into the National Health Service – the lessons of the problems created by the unmanaged introduction of cervical screening seemed to have been learned. This committee was a subcommittee of the Standing Medical Advisory Committee (SMAC) and thus its authority was limited. Its terms of reference were as follows:

1 to review the field of diagnostic screening of the population for disease
2 to identify areas of needed research (co-operating where indicated with other Departmental Advisory Committees)
3 to consider the implications for resources
4 to advise the Standing Medical Advisory Committees of the Secretary of State

for Social Services and the Secretary of State for Scotland (Scottish Health Services Planning Council) on the justification for and operation of screening services.

The first meeting was held in January 1969 and the sub-committee continued until September 1980, when no further meeting was scheduled 'pending SMAC's consideration of the future of the Sub-Committee.'

The National Screening Committee

There was then a planning gap on screening until the United Kingdom National Screening Committee (NSC) was established in 1996 and an effective mechanism was set up – covering the four countries of the UK – both to influence the implementation of effective programmes and to identify areas for further research.

The remit and terms of reference of the NSC are as follows.

1 The UK National Screening Committee will advise Ministers, the devolved national assemblies and the Scottish Parliament on:
   - the case for implementing new population screening programmes not presently purchased by the NHS within each of the countries of the UK
   - screening technologies that are of proven effectiveness but which require controlled and well-managed introduction
   - the case for continuing, modifying or withdrawing existing population screening programmes, in particular programmes that have been inadequately evaluated or which are of doubtful effectiveness, quality or value.
2 The NSC will call on sound evidence to inform its advice and recommendations. In particular this will involve:
   - calling on the advice of the Standing Group on Health Technologies Diagnostic Technologies Panel (formerly the Population Screening Panel), and in turn informing the setting of NHS Research and Development priorities
   - calling on the Department of Health Policy Research Programme and defining research needs for screening
   - calling on other appropriate sources of sound evidence from within and outside the NHS.
3 The NSC will set up practical mechanisms to oversee the introduction of a new programme and its implementation in the NHS. It will monitor effectiveness and quality assurance.
4 The NSC will be informed by reports from the advisory groups for specific programmes on the performance of those programmes and issues that arise which would have relevance to general screening policy.

Thus the NSC has a much more defined role and, by reporting to Ministers, has greater authority than its predecessor, the Joint Standing Sub-Committee. It is responsible for introducing proven screening programmes and for evaluating them, and is thus not merely an advisory body. It also represents an important central reference point for all considerations of screening in the UK although, since screening is a devolved matter, it is theoretically open to each of the four countries to make their own interpretation of the NSC's advice.

Changing definitions and perceptions of screening

In 1968, McKeown[12] defined screening as a 'medical investigation which does not arise from a patient's request for advice for a specific complaint.' Screening thus defined may have one or more of three main aims, and the requirements for its acceptance may be quite different in each case. First, it may be the subject of research – for example, in the validation of a procedure before it is introduced more widely. Secondly, it can be used for the protection of public health (sometimes compulsorily) to identify a source of infection – for example, in the search for the source of an outbreak of food poisoning. Thirdly, screening can have as its main aim a direct contribution to the health of individuals.

There have been various definitions of screening over the years, and a number of the most prominent ones are summarised in Table 1.1.

These definitions do not differ greatly in meaning, although the most recent one from the NSC is hedged round with some rather heavy circumlocution,

Table 1.1 Summary of definitions of screening

Source	Definition
US Commission on Chronic Illness (1957)[6]	Screening is the presumptive identification of unrecognised disease or defect by the application of tests, examinations or other procedures, which can be applied rapidly. Screening tests sort out apparently well persons who apparently have a disease from those who probably do not
McKeown (1968)[12]	Screening is a medical investigation which does not arise from a patient's request for advice for a specific complaint
Wilson and Jungner (1968)[11]	Mass screening is the large-scale screening of whole population groups. Selective screening is the screening of certain high-risk groups in the population. Multiphasic screening is the administration of two or more screening tests to large groups of people. Surveillance is long-term observation of individual populations. Case finding is the screening of patients who are already in contact with the health services to detect disease and start treatment. Early disease detection refers to all types of screening
National Screening Committee – *First Report* (1998)[13]	Screening is the systematic application of test or inquiry to identify individuals at sufficient risk of a specific disorder to warrant further investigation or direct preventive action among persons who have not sought medical attention on account of symptoms of that disorder
National Screening Committee – *Second Report* (2000)[14]	Screening is a public health service in which members of a defined population, who do not necessarily perceive that they are at risk of, or are already affected by, a disease or its complications, are asked a question or offered a test to identify those individuals who are more likely to be helped than harmed by further tests or treatment to reduce the risk of disease or its complications

presumably to minimise the possibility of consequences arising from the growing climate of complaint or litigation. Wald[15] describes it as 'unwieldy and unclear,' and suggests that the Committee would have done better to stay with its original definition.

Put simply, what we are talking about when referring to screening, as indicated at the start of this chapter, is actively seeking to identify a disease or pre-disease condition in people who are presumed and who presume themselves to be healthy. However, it is important also to acknowledge the difference between *population screening* (where groups of people who are thought to be at risk are invited to attend for screening – as in the national programmes for cancer of the breast and cervix) and *opportunistic screening for prevention* or *case finding* (where individuals have sought medical contact for some reason and the opportunity is taken to suggest various other tests, such as the measurement of blood pressure or cholesterol, appropriate to their age and sex). As Getz and colleagues have pointed out, it may be timely to look critically at the whole question of opportunistic screening in the modern context:[16]

> Medical resources are increasingly shifting from making patients better to preventing them from becoming ill. Genetic testing is likely to extend the list of conditions that can be screened for – is it time to stop and consider whom we screen and how we approach it?

Criteria for screening

The basic criteria to be fulfilled before screening for a condition is introduced have been well rehearsed over the years.[1,11, 17–19] They are absolutely fundamental to the integrity of the screening process, and we make no apology for repeating them here.

Appendix C of the NSC's *Second Report*[14] summarises the criteria as follows, taking account of the 'recent more rigorous standards of evidence required to improve effectiveness and the greater concern about the possible adverse effects of healthcare.' The information is also available on the NSC's website.[20]

The condition

- The condition should be an important health problem.
- The epidemiology and natural history of the condition, including development from latent to declared disease, should be adequately understood and there should be a detectable risk factor or disease marker and a latent period or early symptomatic stage.
- All of the cost-effective primary prevention interventions should have been implemented as far as is practicable.

The test

- There should be a simple, safe, precise and validated screening test.
- The distribution of test values in the target population should be known, and a suitable cut-off level should be defined and agreed.

- The test should be acceptable to the population.
- There should be an agreed policy on the further diagnostic investigation of individuals with a positive test result, and on the choices available to those individuals.

The treatment

- There should be an effective treatment or intervention for patients identified through early detection, with evidence of early treatment leading to better outcomes than late treatment.
- There should be agreed evidence-based policies covering which individuals should be offered treatment and the appropriate treatment to be offered.
- Clinical management of the condition and patient outcomes should be optimised by all healthcare providers prior to participation in a screening programme.
- There must be evidence from high-quality randomised controlled trials that the screening programme is effective in reducing mortality or morbidity. Where screening is aimed solely at providing information to allow the person being screened to make an 'informed choice'(e.g. Down's syndrome or cystic fibrosis carrier screening), there must be evidence from high-quality trials that the test measures risk accurately. The information that is provided about the test and its outcome must be of value and readily understood by the individual who is being screened.
- There should be evidence that the complete screening programme (test, diagnostic procedures and treatment/intervention) is clinically, socially and ethically acceptable to healthcare professionals and the public.
- The benefit from the screening programme should outweigh the physical and psychological harm (caused by the test, diagnostic procedures and treatment).
- The opportunity cost of the screening programme (including testing, diagnosis, treatment, administration, training and quality assurance) should be economically balanced in relation to expenditure on medical care as a whole (i.e. value for money).
- There must be a plan for managing and monitoring the screening programme and an agreed set of quality assurance standards.
- Adequate staffing and facilities for testing, diagnosis, treatment and programme management should be made available prior to the commencement of the screening programme.
- All other options for managing the condition should have been considered (e.g. improving treatment, providing other services) to ensure that no more cost-effective intervention could be introduced or current interventions increased within the resources available.
- Evidence-based information that explains the consequences of testing, investigation and treatment should be made available to potential participants to assist them in making an informed choice.
- Public pressure for widening the eligibility criteria for reducing the screening interval, and for increasing the sensitivity of the testing process, should be anticipated. Decisions about these parameters should be scientifically justifiable to the public.

In less elaborate language, the principles can be grouped into four categories as summarised in Table 1.2.[1]

Table 1.2 Summary of criteria for screening

Category	Criteria
Condition	The condition sought should be an important health problem whose natural history, including development from latent to declared disease, is adequately understood. The condition should have a recognisable latent or early symptomatic stage
Diagnosis	There should be a suitable diagnostic test that is available, safe and acceptable to the population concerned. There should be an agreed policy, based on respectable test findings and national standards, as to whom to regard as patients, and the whole process should be a continuing one
Treatment	There should be an accepted and established treatment or intervention for individuals identified as having the disease or pre-disease condition, and facilities for treatment should be available
Cost	The cost of case finding (including diagnosis and treatment) should be economically balanced in relation to possible expenditure on medical care as a whole

Evaluation of screening

As well as restating the principles that must underlie any reputable screening programme, it is important to emphasise the necessity for scientific evaluation and effective quality control, which we will look at in greater detail in Chapter 3. In the early days of screening, the natural history of the conditions being sought – such as tuberculosis and syphilis – was well understood and lines of treatment were clear. However, with diseases such as HIV/AIDS and a growing emphasis on

Table 1.3 Summary of criteria for evaluation of screening

Factor	Criteria
Simplicity	The test should be simple to perform, easy to interpret and, where possible, capable of use by paramedical and other personnel
Acceptability	Since participation in screening is voluntary, the test must be acceptable to those undergoing it
Accuracy	The test must give a true measurement of the condition or symptom under investigation
Cost	The expense of the test must be considered in relation to the benefits of early detection of the disease
Repeatability	The test should give consistent results in repeated trials
Sensitivity	The test should be capable of giving a positive finding when the individual being screened has the condition being sought
Specificity	The test should be capable of giving a negative finding when the individual being screened does not have the condition being sought

chronic diseases that can take many years to develop and where aetiologies and current treatments may be less certain, the situation is altogether more complex. In 1971, Cochrane and Holland suggested seven criteria for evaluation. These have stood the test of time (*see* Table 1.3).[17]

Political issues and public perceptions

In recent years screening has taken on a far higher profile than was previously the case, and has become a politically sensitive issue. There are a number of forces at work here.

First, people have become increasingly knowledgeable about health matters as a result of media focus and the wide availability of health-related information, of whatever quality, on the Internet. There is thus a popular demand for more effective healthcare and the firm belief, among many, that early diagnosis provided by screening will inevitably lead to a better outcome. This demand is being fuelled by charities such as those concerned with cancer, who believe that screening can only be beneficial. Private clinics and healthcare providers advertise general screening programmes for men and women – a human version of the MOT.† Pressure and lay groups, together with the media, may excite a public demand for screening for a particular condition on the basis of a specific case, unsupported by scientific evidence with regard to its efficacy. There is also the possibility of well-intentioned doctors, patients and pressure groups leading a virtual crusade against a particular disease or group of diseases and persuading governments to provide a screening programme before a proper assessment of benefit is available.

Secondly, screening has become a commercial enterprise – not only in terms of the promotion and performance of the procedures, but also in terms of the supply of equipment and reagents. Thus part of the process is driven by financial interests. Examples of this include private mobile units sited in supermarket car parks providing some appropriate tests, such as screening for cancers of the breast and cervix. However, many other tests that are offered do not conform to accepted criteria and are not linked to a system that monitors the results and identifies individuals at greatest risk.

Thirdly, governments are willing to invest in screening services even at high cost and with relatively small benefits (e.g. screening for cancer of the breast) in order to demonstrate that they are concerned with the provision of services that improve health in general and prevention in particular. The NSC's remit and terms of reference include the statement that it will advise on 'the case for continuing, modifying or withdrawing existing population programmes.' Despite this, one politician did actually suggest to us that any government would be most unlikely to halt an existing screening service even if there was good scientific evidence that there was no benefit (personal communication, 2002).

Finally, despite the increased demand for screening, there has been a drop in public confidence. In the past decade there has been at least one annual 'scandal' because of deficiencies in the provision of screening services, mainly those for cervical cancer. Because of the large numbers of smears examined, errors are

---

† The MOT is an annual test of roadworthiness required in the UK for any car over three years old.

bound to occur in this and in any screening programme. The concepts of false positives and false negatives are difficult to understand, and the media are not slow to highlight – and, indeed, to dramatise – problems of inadequate staffing and training or lapses in administrative efficiency, as well as incompetence by a few professionals. Screening in itself is not a guarantee of diagnosis and cure, but rather it is one tool in the prevention of disease.

As the *Second Report* of the NSC points out, 'errors occur in all branches of medicine and are inevitable.'[14] In the clinical care of individual patients, adverse events come to the attention of the public and the media in a sporadic way, spread across many clinical specialties. In a national screening programme involving large numbers of women and subject to stringent quality control, such as that for cervical cancer, errors and problems quickly become public knowledge. Steps have to be taken to restore public confidence in screening and to better inform the public and the media of the nature of screening and its merits and limitations.

Increased political involvement and interest in screening are exemplified by a conference on parliaments and screening, with particular reference to ethical and social problems arising from testing and screening for HIV and AIDS, held in 1995 in the European Parliament.[21]

In a PhD thesis entitled 'The Politics of Breast Cancer Screening,' published in 1996, Hann took a feminist viewpoint in which she criticised the Forrest Report that recommended the introduction of a national programme in the UK.[22] She suggested that the members of the Working Party which produced the Report had been chosen for their views on the benefits of the scheme without sufficient balance from an alternative standpoint.

The Council of Europe has also commented on the need to develop screening services on the basis of clear principles and criteria in a recommendation to the Committee of Ministers on screening as a tool in preventive medicine.[23] This document also emphasises the possible adverse effects of screening, which can include:

- stigmatisation and/or discrimination of (non-)participants
- social pressure to participate in the screening and undergo the intended treatment/intervention
- psychological distress in cases where there is no cure for the disease or where the treatment and/or intervention is morally unacceptable to the individual concerned
- exposure to physical and psychological risks with limited health gains
- creation of expectations which probably cannot be fulfilled
- individuals who are positively screened possibly experiencing difficulties such as access to insurance, employment, etc.
- severe side-effects of invasive clinical diagnosis of false positives
- delay in diagnosing false negatives
- the unfavourable cost–benefit relationship of a screening programme.

This paper also raises important legal and ethical issues. For example, it stresses that although effectiveness is a necessary prerequisite for the screening to be ethical, screening can be effective and still unethical. We shall look more closely at the ethics of screening in Chapter 3.

The involvement of the state in screening is also well illustrated in China, where a premarital examination for hereditary illnesses and psychiatric problems which could jeopardise parenting abilities is mandatory.[24] This is the most extreme form of screening that we have encountered. Although some of the conditions identified (e.g. sexually transmitted diseases, tuberculosis and phimosis) might be treatable, the ethical implications of such a mandatory examination are enormous and, of course, of particular consequence with the development of genetic screening.

Benefit or bane?

Views on the value of screening continue to vary. Screening still has its evangelists and its agnostics, and there is little doubt that the latter group has grown – at least among healthcare professionals – in recent years.

In 1988, Skrabanek restated his view that 'screening healthy people without informing them about the magnitude of inherent risks of screening is ethically unjustifiable.'[25] Screening differs from traditional medical practice in that it aims to detect disease at a very early stage, either before or very soon after symptoms present, and sometimes before an individual decides to seek medical advice. It therefore carries very considerable ethical responsibilities, as it has the potential to transform individuals from a state of supposing themselves to be healthy to a state of having some disorder or potential disorder. Screening should not be used to identify conditions that are either insignificant or untreatable, since at either end of that spectrum lie anxiety and anguish. As Wald and Cuckle stated in 1989,[26] 'Screening must be principally concerned with the prevention of disease and the recognition that it is only worthwhile screening for disorders which lend themselves to effective intervention.' This is well worth re-emphasising today.

An editorial in the *British Medical Journal* in 2003 examined the modern screening industry.[27] With the advent of whole-body scans, the marketing of health has intensified. The sales pitch is simple and on the surface beguiling. You may have some disease or abnormality lurking in your system. Either the scan will show it and allow early treatment, or it will give you the all-clear and you can then celebrate.

In the same issue of the *British Medical Journal*, Swensen describes his experience of using computed tomography to screen for lung cancer within the context of a major clinical trial.[28] His research team found 700 ancillary findings within its cohort, but most were false positives which led to adversely affected quality of life and unnecessary diagnostic and interventional procedures. And Raffle and colleagues, in a study of screening for cervical cancer, showed that 1000 women have to be screened for 35 years to prevent one death from the disease.[29]

The editorial concluded:[27]

> Simple-minded enthusiasm for screening – combined with industrial opportunity to make fat profits – may mean that soon none of us will be normal. . . . It's always hard to put the case for 'not knowing,' but economists . . . have a wonderful notion of 'rational ignorance.' It simply isn't sensible to try to know everything. Ignorance can be bliss.

Another issue that deserves attention was raised by Muir Gray,[30] who argued that screening is a programme, not a test. This is one of the problems that the health service has with private sector screening, where an individual may be offered a test for a specific condition but the investigation and reassurance for those who test positive are then passed to the National Health Service even though the condition tested for did not meet the NHS screening criteria (e.g. ovarian or prostate cancer).

There is a need for balance in the screening debate, and that must surely lie between the extremes of enthusiasm and doubt in a cautious and rigorous consideration of all screening practices and proposals. As Russell[31] has described, there is a growing body of research indicating that the chronic degenerative diseases of middle or old age can often be prevented or at least delayed, and new vaccines can also offer better protection against infectious diseases. Such developments offer the prospect of better ways to maintain health and prolong life, and have led to a new surge of interest in preventive activities such as screening. The question that must be asked of any preventive measure, or indeed of any investment in health, is whether the gains in health are a reasonable return for the risks and costs involved.

Sackett[32] calls time on the arrogance of preventive medicine and emphasises that the 'fundamental promise we make when we actively solicit individuals and exhort them to accept preventive interventions must be that, on average, they will be the better for it.' He cites the example of the Women's Health Initiative randomised controlled trial of hormone replacement therapy, which was stopped when it became clear that the participating women's risk of cardiovascular disease increased rather than decreased on active therapy:[33] 'Without evidence from randomised trials (and, better still, systematic reviews of randomised trials) we cannot justify soliciting the well to accept any personal health intervention.'

Twenty years ago, Chamberlain[34] summarised the benefits and disadvantages of screening, and her analysis remains valid today (*see* Table 1.4).

The benefits are straightforward. Early accurate diagnosis and intervention will lead to an improved prognosis in some patients. At this stage treatment may need to be less radical. Scarce health services resources will be conserved by treating diseases before they progress, and patients with true negative test results can be reassured.

Table 1.4 Benefits and disadvantages of screening

Benefits	Disadvantages
Improved prognosis for some cases detected	Longer morbidity for cases whose prognosis is unaltered
Less radical treatment which cures some early cases	Overtreatment of questionable abnormalities
Resource savings	Resource costs
Reassurance for those with negative test results	False reassurance for those with false-negative results
	Anxiety and sometimes morbidity for those with false-positive results
	Hazard of screening test itself

Source: Chamberlain.[34] Reproduced by kind permission of the author and the publisher.

The disadvantages are more complicated. There will be longer periods of morbidity for patients whose prognosis is unchanged, and there may be over-treatment of non-serious conditions or abnormalities identified and individuals may become anxious. Haynes and colleagues found an increase in absenteeism from work in steelworkers with raised diastolic pressure after they had been given the diagnosis:[35] 'The increase in illness absenteeism bears a striking relationship to the employee's awareness of the diagnosis, but appears unaffected by the institution of antihypertensive therapy or the degree of success in reducing blood pressure.'

Work by Marteau and colleagues[36-39] and Austoker[40] has confirmed the problems of anxiety induced by screening, and these will be discussed more fully later in the book in terms both of antenatal and adult screening.

There are also resource costs involved in finding more illness, in terms of the tests themselves, the personnel costs and the subsequent management of whatever is found. There is the unpalatable certainty that some individuals with false-negative results will be given unfounded reassurance and that those with false-positive results will experience at the very least unnecessary anxiety and at the worst inappropriate treatment. Finally there is the possibility, however remote, of hazard from the screening test itself.

Austoker quotes from one of the conclusions of a report on cervical screening in Bristol: 'by offering screening to 250 000 we have helped a few, harmed thousands, disappointed many, used £1.5million each year, and kept a few lawyers in work.'[40] She emphasises the importance of obtaining truly informed consent for screening and of respecting the patient's autonomy, including their right to decide not to undergo a screening procedure.

The present monograph

Our plan for this book has been to devote Chapters 1, 2 and 3 to a general overview of screening and its history and some of the key issues that it involves. In subsequent chapters we follow a life-cycle approach in four screening segments as summarised in Table 1.5. Chapter 8 contains a brief account of screening practices in Europe, and the final chapter provides an overview and looks cautiously into the future.

When we began to plan the writing we expected to find that many changes had occurred since the publication of the first edition in 1990. However, the general principles and criteria have stood the test of time, and although much knowledge

Table 1.5 Life-cycle screening segments

Segment	Stage of life	Age range (years)
I	Antenatal, neonatal, infancy	< 1
II	Childhood	1–11
	Adolescence and early adulthood	12–24
III	Adulthood	25–64
IV	The elderly	≥ 65

and experience have accumulated, particularly in the field of human genetics, few dramatic new issues have emerged.

The main changes have been first in emphasis and secondly in increased politicisation.

Fifteen years ago there was great enthusiasm for screening among many healthcare professionals. That has been largely replaced by a more cautious approach and a more open acknowledgement that screening can also cause harm.

Politicians meanwhile – perhaps reflecting popular opinion – have become far more convinced of the need for screening services, but have also on occasion been over-ready to attribute blame for the inevitable mistakes and shortcomings to those providing the service. Screening must not become a political tool that is used to convince the public of action in an increasingly beleaguered health service.

The establishment of the National Screening Committee has provided a very valuable focus and point of reference for screening activities, and the NSC is now able to advise Ministers on screening for various conditions on the basis of sound evidence. It has also highlighted two themes that will underpin its working over the next decade – those of *informed choice* and *risk reduction* – so that people can make their own decisions as to whether or not to participate in a particular programme within the context of a clear understanding of what screening can and cannot offer.

The book is not intended as a comprehensive review of screening for specialists in a particular branch of medicine. Rather, we have tried to take a general look at screening, to discuss some of the important ethical, economic and quality issues involved, to review current practice in screening at the various stages of life, and finally to suggest some constructive ways forward.

We hope that the book will be of interest and value to healthcare professionals across the field – from medicine to management – to medical, nursing and other health-related students and to anyone seeking to understand what screening is really about.

Screening covers the entire lifespan, from before conception to old age. It can never be perfect but, used wisely, it can be a potent force for health improvement in the twenty-first century.

References

1 Holland WW and Stewart S (1990) *Screening in Healthcare*. The Nuffield Provincial Hospitals Trust, London.

2 Hawthorne VM (1964) Mass radiography in an ecological approach to respiratory disease. *Scott Med J.* **9**: 115–24.

3 Semple A (1953, 1960, 1966) *Annual Reports for the City of Liverpool.*

4 Godber GE (1986) Medical Officers of Health and Health Services. *Commun Med.* **8**: 114.

5 Breslow L and Roberts DW (eds) (1955) Screening for asymptomatic disease. *J Chron Dis.* **2**: 363–490.

6 Commission on Chronic Illness (1957) *Chronic Illness in the USA. Volume I. Prevention of chronic illness.* Harvard University Press, Cambridge, MA.

7 Thorner RM and Remein QR (1961) *Principles and Procedures in the Evaluation of Screening for Disease.* PHS publication no. 846. Public Health Monograph no 67. Public Health Service, Washington, DC.

8 Ahluwahlia HS and Doll R (1968) Mortality from cancer of the cervix uteri in British Columbia and other parts of Canada. *Br J Prev Soc Med.* **22:** 161–4.

9 Collen MF (1988) *History of the Kaiser Permanente Medical Care Program.* An interview conducted by Sally Smith Hughes. Regional Oral History Office, Bancroft Library, University of California, Berkeley, CA.

10 Godber GE (1975) *The Health Service Past, Present and Future.* Athlone Press, London.

11 Wilson JMG and Jungner G (1968) *Principles and Practice of Screening for Disease.* World Health Organization, Geneva.

12 McKeown T (ed.) (1968) *Screening in Medical Care: reviewing the evidence.* Oxford University Press for the Nuffield Provincial Hospitals Trust, Oxford.

13 Health Departments of the United Kingdom (1998) *First Report of the UK National Screening Committee.* Health Departments of the United Kingdom, London.

14 Health Departments of the United Kingdom (2000) *Second Report of the UK National Screening Committee.* Health Departments of the United Kingdom, London.

15 Wald NJ (2001) The definition of screening (editorial). *J Med Screen.* **8:** 1.

16 Getz L, Sigurdsson JA and Hetlevik I (2003) Is opportunistic disease prevention in the consultation ethically justifiable? *BMJ.* **327:** 498–500.

17 Cochrane AL and Holland WW (1971) Validation of screening procedures. *Br Med Bull.* **27:** 3–8.

18 Cuckle HS and Wald NJ (1984) Principles of screening. In: NJ Wald (ed.) *Antenatal and Neonatal Screening.* Oxford University Press, Oxford.

19 Gray JAM (1996) *Dimensions and Definitions of Screening.* NHS Executive Anglia and Oxford, Research and Development Directorate, Milton Keynes.

20 www.nsc.nhs.uk/

21 Wayland K (ed.) (1995) *Parliaments and Screening. A conference on the ethical and social problems arising from testing and screening for HIV and AIDS: the role of parliaments and the media. Conference Report and studies of the handling of bioethics in the 12 national parliaments of the European Union.* John Libbey Eurotext, Paris.

22 Hann A (1996) *The Politics of Breast Cancer Screening.* Avebury, Aldershot.

23 Council of Europe (1994) Recommendation No R(94)11 on screening as a tool of preventive medicine; www.coe.int/T/E/Social_Cohesion/Health/Recommendations/Rec(1994)11.asp

24 Hesketh T (2003) Getting married in China: pass the medical first. *BMJ.* **326:** 277–9.

25 Skrabanek P (1988) The physician's responsibility to the patient. *Lancet.* **1:** 1155–7.

26 Wald N and Cuckle H (1989) Reporting the assessment of screening and diagnostic tests. *Br J Obstet Gynaecol.* **96:** 389–96.

27 Smith R (2003) The screening industry (editorial). *BMJ.* **326:** 891.

28 Swensen SJ (2003) Screening for cancer with computed tomography (editorial). *BMJ.* **326:** 894–5.

29 Raffle AE, Alden B, Quinn M, Babb J and Brett MT (2003) Outcomes of screening to prevent cancer: analysis of cumulative incidence of cervical abnormality and modelling of cases and deaths prevented. *BMJ.* **326:** 901–9.

30 Muir Gray JA (2004) New concepts in screening. *Br J Gen Pract.* **54:** 292–8.

31 Russell LB (1986) *Is Prevention Better than Cure?* The Brookings Institute, Washington, DC.

32 Sackett D (2002) The arrogance of preventive medicine. *Can Med Assoc J.* **167:** 363–5.

33 Writing Group for the Women's Health Initiative Investigators (2002) Risks and benefits of estrogen plus progestin in healthy postmenopausal women. Principal results from the Women's Health Initiative randomised controlled trial. *JAMA.* **288:** 321–33.

34 Chamberlain JM (1984) Which prescriptive screening programmes are worthwhile? *J Epidemiol Commun Health.* **38:** 270–77.

35 Haynes RB, Sackett DL, Taylor DW, Gibson ES and Johnson AL (1978) Increased absenteeism from work after detection and labelling of hypertensive patients. *NEJM.* **299:** 741–4.

36 Marteau TM, Cook R, Kidd J *et al.* (1992) The psychological effects of false-positive results in prenatal screening for fetal abnormality: a prospective study. *Prenat Diagn.* **12:** 205–14.

37 Marteau TM, Slack J, Kidd J and Shaw RW (1992) Presenting a routine screening test in antenatal care: practice observed. *Public Health.* **106:** 131–41.

38 Marteau TM, Kidd J, Michie S, Cook R, Johnston M and Shaw RW (1993) Anxiety, knowledge and satisfaction in women receiving false-positive results on routine prenatal screening: a randomised controlled trial. *J Psychometr Obstet Gynaecol.* **14:** 185–96.

39 Shaw RW, Abrams K and Marteau TM (1999) Psychological impact of predicting individuals' risks of illness: a systematic review. *Soc Sci Med.* **49:** 1571–98.

40 Austoker J (1999) Gaining informed consent for screening (editorial). *BMJ.* **319:** 722–3.

Chapter 2

Key issues in screening: genetics, information and economics

> Genetic technologies have the potential to be of major benefit to mankind, but their introduction must be measured, attentive to the social and ethical considerations of the day, and, most importantly, based on best evidence.*

Introduction

The key issues discussed in this chapter and in Chapter 3 are fundamental at all stages and in every type of screening, and are closely interrelated. Genetic screening is an area that has developed rapidly in recent years with the mapping of the human genome. Information that is balanced, understandable and properly communicated to those invited to undergo screening in any context is an essential part of obtaining truly informed consent. And the economics of screening must be examined in a health service where demand, whether justified or unjustified, is always going to exceed available resources, since these tests and the treatment or follow-up that may be needed usually require a great deal of resources – human, technical and financial.

Genetic screening

Developments in genetics in recent years have opened up many new possibilities for the diagnosis of a variety of diseases, and have been considered by many to herald a new era in the prevention, early diagnosis or identification of disease.

The central issue in genetic screening – by which we mean the identification of inherited disorders that have significant consequences for the individual and/or family members – is whether there is anything distinctive in this process compared with other forms of non-genetic screening. We believe that the same principles apply to genetic screening as to any other form of screening – that is, if genetic screening is offered to any individual, either there must be an effective intervention available for anyone found to be affected, or the information provided by the result must help the individual and other family members to make better decisions than if the information was not available.

There are a number of instances where genetic screening may be helpful. For example, a child known to have multiple endocrine neoplasia type 2 (MEN-2) can be spared medullary carcinoma by undergoing prophylactic thyroidectomy, or an adult with hereditary haemochromatosis can avoid cirrhosis by the early initiation of phlebotomy treatment.

* Melzer M and Zimmern R (2002) Genetics and medicalisation. *BMJ.* **324**: 863–4.

Genetic tests

A genetic test is 'the analysis of human DNA, RNA, chromosomes, proteins and certain metabolites in order to detect heritable disease-related genotypes, mutations, phenotypes or karyotypes for clinical purposes.'[1] As Burke[2] has stated, this definition reflects the broad range of techniques used in the testing process. A comprehensive and constantly updated list of currently available tests can be found at the GeneTests-GeneClinics website.[3]

For example, genetic tests can be used in Duchenne's muscular dystrophy (in which both molecular and biochemical tests are used), sickle-cell anaemia (in which both molecular and haematological tests are used) and breast and ovarian cancers (where molecular, panel and sequencing tests are used). Molecular genetic tests can be used, for instance, for Huntington's disease, β-thalassaemia and α-antitrypsin deficiency.

This is not the place to describe the methodology used for the wide variety of genetic tests now available, and full information on this subject may be found at the website mentioned above. It is essential to obtain a family history before genetic tests are considered, since this illuminates both the likely risk and the type of test required, and to appreciate that the results may be of huge significance to the extended family of the individual tested.

Genetic screening can help in evaluating risk, but if little can be done to alter the finding, the need for and use of such information has to be considered extremely carefully. A good example of this is testing for Huntington's disease, an autosomal dominant condition that causes progressive motor and cognitive dysfunction starting in midlife. Genetic testing would allow individuals with an affected parent to determine whether they have inherited the causative mutation. However, if the latter is present, the individual's risk of developing Huntington's disease is virtually 100% and no effective prevention or treatment is available.

A recent *British Medical Journal* news item reported that a young teacher in Germany was refused a permanent job on the grounds that members of her family had Huntington's disease, and that she was therefore at risk of developing the condition.[4] The decision of the education authority in question was condemned by the chairman of the German National Ethics Council. He observed that no one has any guarantees about their future health, and if the government was prepared to accept the risk that employees might develop alcoholism, depression or other forms of ill health – as it does – then it should also accept the risks associated with genetic diseases.

In the case of X-linked recessive conditions such as Duchenne muscular dystrophy, the purpose of genetic testing is to identify family members who are carriers (those who are themselves unaffected but are at risk of having affected children). As with Huntington's disease, no prevention or treatment is available, but identification of the risk will enable people to make appropriate decisions.

However, as Stone and Stewart have pointed out,[5] the two most frequently cited objectives of screening for a recessive carrier state are to reduce the prevalence of the disorder and to inform the reproductive choices of individuals and couples at risk: 'The latter aim represents a paradigm shift in the philosophy of screening in that no preventive principle is involved. Instead information is regarded as worthwhile in itself, regardless of outcome.' These authors go on to suggest that the benefits that arise from the information generated in the course of genetic carrier screening cannot be presumed merely by asserting a 'right to know' ethical imperative, and they draw attention to the danger that a combination of technical capability, professional zeal and consumer demand may override long-established screening principles.

Uses of genetic screening

Genetic screening can be used in a variety of settings for a number of purposes.

- *Diagnostic testing* is used to confirm or exclude a suspected genetic disorder in an asymptomatic individual.
- *Predictive testing* is used in individuals who are asymptomatic but have a family history of a genetic disorder. It may be:
  - presymptomatic, when the gene mutation is present (e.g. Huntington's disease)
  - predispositional, when eventual development of symptoms is possible but not certain (e.g. breast cancer).

Predictive testing is indicated if early diagnosis allows an intervention that reduces morbidity or mortality and can influence life-planning decisions. Because predictive testing is so problematic, particularly in the absence of effective interventions, even if it enhances the ability of individuals to make informed decisions, it is essential that key prerequisites are met. Adequate information about the test and its interpretation must be given to the individuals concerned, and there must be evidence that they have understood this information. Genetic counselling services must be made available. In general, identification of the specific gene mutation in an affected relative or establishment of linkage within the family should precede predictive testing. As Ridley has stated in a discussion of Huntington's disease, 'Nothing is more sensitive than the results of a test for a fatal disease; telling people starkly and coldly may well not be the best thing to do – for them. Testing without counselling is a recipe for misery.'[6]

- *Carrier testing* is performed in order to identify individuals who have a gene mutation for a disorder inherited in an autosomal recessive or X-linked manner. Carriers normally have no symptoms related to the gene mutation. This type of testing is usually undertaken in individuals who have family members with a genetic condition, in family members of an identified carrier, or in members of an ethnic or racial group known to have a higher than normal carrier rate for a particular condition. It is thus a method of screening a high-risk group to enable individuals to make properly informed choices about reproductive and other issues.
- *Prenatal testing* may be used in cases where there is thought to be an increased risk of an affected fetus because of maternal age, family history, ethnicity, biochemical tests or fetal ultrasound findings. The usual tests are amniocentesis and chorionic villus sampling. More specialised procedures include placental biopsy, periumbilical blood sampling and fetoscopy with fetal skin biopsy. All prenatal genetic diagnostic tests carry risks and may result in fetal loss.
- *Pre-implantation testing* is undertaken on early embryos after *in-vitro* fertilisation to minimise the risk of a genetic condition in couples at particular risk. It is not an easy procedure and is only performed in a few specialised centres. It is also

technically demanding both because of the difficulty in obtaining eggs and also because of problems with DNA analysis.

- *Newborn screening* aims to identify affected individuals at as early a stage as possible in order to start treatment (e.g. by detecting cystic fibrosis or sickle-cell disease).

- *Preventive screening* – in a number of common conditions, genetic tests may contribute to the identification of individuals at particularly high risk. For example, testing for BRCA1 and BRCA2 mutations can identify women at high risk from breast cancer, although these mutations are rare. Of '10 000 women, 1000 will have a mother or sister who has had breast cancer, but only 15 will have a mutation that confers a high risk. It is estimated that in a primary care practice of 1000 patients, one case of inherited breast cancer will be diagnosed every one to two years, but one case of inherited breast cancer caused by BRCA1 or BRCA2 mutation will be diagnosed every 20 years.'[7] Estimates of lifetime risk of breast cancers associated with these mutations range from 26% to 85%.[8] This has not stopped some women from demanding these tests and then, if they prove positive, undergoing prophylactic mastectomies.

As Burke[2] emphasises, this is only a start. The Human Genome Project will enable tests to be developed to identify variants, probably of lower risk, that contribute to many common conditions such as cardiovascular disease or various forms of cancer. This will present a major challenge because the tests are likely to have a larger proportion of false negatives and false positives as well as being technically far more complex than more routine screening tests. The ability to identify genetic markers will certainly outpace the ability to provide effective treatments. Ridley has drawn attention to the 'uselessness of diagnosing without curing.'[6]

Problems of genetic screening

The identification of the human genome and the rapid development of a variety of biochemical and molecular genetic tests have raised the expectations of the public as well as those of scientists and doctors about the possible contributions that such knowledge may provide in the prevention and cure of many diseases. These expectations must be tempered by considering some of the pitfalls and problems.

In this discussion we are not concerned with the use of genetic tests to improve diagnosis (and treatment) of a known condition. Rather we are concerned with the tests for recessive carrier states in the population, such as that for deletion in the dystrophin gene, the cause of Duchenne's muscular dystrophy, which can be used to identify women who are carriers of the condition. These women can thus avoid pregnancy or undergo prenatal testing for Duchenne's muscular dystrophy, with possible pregnancy termination if the fetus is found to be affected.

On a general level, Ridley is among those who have drawn attention to the tendency to define genes by the diseases that they cause: 'Open any catalogue of the human genome and you will be confronted not with a list of human potentialities but a list of diseases. . . . The impression given is that genes are there to cause diseases . . . new gene for mental illness . . . gene for early-onset dystonia . . . gene for kidney cancer isolated.'[6] He contends that this is about as absurd as defining organs of the body by the disease they get: 'Livers are there to cause cirrhosis, hearts to cause heart attacks and brains to cause strokes. It is a measure not of our knowledge, but of our ignorance, that this is the way the genome catalogues read.'

Colhoun and colleagues have recently summarised the major difficulties in the interpretation of genetic associations reported in complex diseases.[9] The human genome has several million single-nucleotide polymorphisms and thus 'the number of possible genetic associations is limited only by the rate at which laboratories are able to type these polymorphisms.' Furthermore, published reports of significant associations can only rarely be replicated. We are thus faced with the common epidemiological problem of the interpretation of studies of an association in selected samples of a population. Starting from the question 'Is the association study strategy futile?' these workers describe the problems in detail and conclude that:

> consensus between scientists and journal editors is needed about better ways to interpret and manage data emerging from genetic association studies so we can reduce the number of spurious findings that are declared significant and allow all available data to be collated without bias.[9]

As with all screening tests, genetic tests may also have psychological consequences. Broadstock and colleagues undertook a systematic review of published papers which used standardised outcome measures in genetic tests for Huntington's disease, hereditary breast and ovarian cancer, familial adenomatous polyposis and spinocerebellar ataxia.[10] Although none of the studies reported increased distress in carriers or non-carriers at any point over a 12-month period, all of them were of self-selected populations who agreed to participate in psychological studies. The authors emphasise that most predictive genetic testing is currently being offered within research programmes: 'As genetic testing is diffused from this academic context into routine clinical practice, some of the protective factors associated with the research environment are likely to be reduced. Higher rates of adverse consequences for those tested may occur.'[10] They see an urgent need for further empirical studies, in particular on the relationship between counselling and emotional outcome.

Some of the concerns of those undergoing genetic screening tests have been described in a systematic study of screening for Huntington's disease.[11,12] Data were collected on all pre-symptomatic genetic tests for Huntington's disease in the UK, comprising 2937 completed tests over a 10-year period. Of these, 91% of subjects were at 50% prior risk and 41% of the tests were reported as abnormal or high risk. In South Wales, semi-structured interviews were conducted with 22 test applicants who requested predictive testing, as well as with 32 non-requesters drawn from the South Wales Huntington's disease register.

This study illustrated the difficulties in communication within families and the uncertainties inherent in being at risk and undergoing testing. Important factors in the decision to undergo predictive tests included moral imperatives to clarify one's genetic status, views about the controllability of the future, family attitudes and norms, and the impact of a test result on the family. Even if predictive screening is feasible, therefore, it is crucial that it is adequately and sensitively discussed with those who are invited to be tested. No universal prescription for this process can be given, as it will be dependent on the norms and attitudes of the population from whom the subjects are drawn. Many of those at risk from Huntington's disease, who since 1986 have been eligible to be tested for the mutation, have chosen ignorance.

Melzer and Zimmern[13] have drawn attention to a further danger. Population expectations of genetic screening are enormous, fuelled by the ability to identify a few rare conditions such as Huntington's disease. However, most common conditions are the result of a complex of behavioural and environmental factors in combination with some biological and genetic factors. The emphasis on the latter and the expectations of the population that magic therapeutic bullets will be able to provide solutions may lead to neglect of far more important factors, such as smoking, dirty water or environmental carcinogens. This, as Holtzman[14] points out, leads to the demand for (and provision of) genetic testing of workers for predisposition due to harmful workplace exposures that are very rare, and neglect of the far greater benefits to most workers of simply cleaning up the workplace.

As Burke and colleagues (among others) have stated, it has been rare for publications that deal with genetic screening to have addressed the principles of screening.[15] They often neglect to address such issues as informed consent, adequacy of scientific evidence, balance of risks and benefits, costs and resources used, predictive power of the tests, efficacy of intervention, social consequences of testing and quality control of the tests used. Thus in many instances important ethical principles are neglected.[16]

These ethical issues have been raised cogently by members of disability rights movements, who argue that genetic screening does not share:

> the traditional medical goal of preventing or treating disease in individuals, but instead seeks to prevent the existence of people with disabilities. Prenatal screening has the goal of identifying potential parents at risk of genetically passing on serious disease or identifying an affected fetus so that the pregnancy can be terminated. This is criticised as eugenic . . . rather than providing therapy.[17]

These arguments do need to be debated, although genetic screening to prevent serious disease is considered by many to be a legitimate public health goal.

Possibilities for the application of genetic screening

When we consider the place of genetic screening in the provision of screening services, some fundamentals need to be appreciated, as Vineis and colleagues have emphasised.[18]

1 Gene–environment interactions are intrinsic in the mode of action of low-penetrance genes.
2 Only highly penetrant (i.e. highly deleterious) mutations in cancer genes may act with no interactions with external factors.
3 The relationship between the frequency of a variant and its penetrance is almost inverse – the more penetrant a mutation is, the less frequent it is in the population.
4 The proportion of diseases attributable to specific low-penetrance genetic traits is probably much lower than the burden of disease attributable to certain environmental agents.

5 To credit genes with a major independent role in the courses of complex diseases constitutes scientific misjudgement of the way that genetics affects disease risk.

6 To assess the role of a gene–environment interaction and screening in a population we need to know the penetrance of the genetic trait and its frequency.

7 A useful approach is to combine penetrance and frequency by computing the number needed to screen in order to prevent one case of a target disease.

8 A reasonable (i.e. low) number needed to screen is achieved only by screening for highly penetrant mutations in high-risk families, not by screening for such mutations in the general population or for low-penetrance polymorphisms.

The conclusion must be that genetic population screening is usually not the best option, although a recent study from Iran suggests that it can be used to prevent thalassaemia in that particular population.[19] The focus should normally be on screening high-risk groups and individuals for a few clearly defined conditions.

To illustrate the limited possibilities, Tryggvadøttir has listed possible candidates for such screening in cancer.[20] He groups the conditions as those where a result will change medical care (familial adenomatous polyposis, multiple endocrine neoplasia 2a and 2b, retinoblastoma and von Hippel–Lindau syndrome) and those where identification is less likely to lead to clinical benefit (hereditary non-polyposis colon cancer, hereditary breast and ovarian cancer and Li-Fraumeni syndrome).

It is absolutely essential to accept and to place in context the limited possibilities of the enormously publicised developments of the human genome:

> Some time in the 1970s . . . the old world of certainty, stability and determinism in biology fell. In its place we must build a world of fluctuation, change and unpredictability. The genome that we decipher in this generation is but a snapshot of an ever-changing document. There is no definitive edition.[20]

Information

The importance of information permeates this book in general terms as well as in specific contexts. Few would disagree that clear information about the benefits and harms of any screening procedure should be available to all individuals invited to participate in any programme. In practice, however, it is not enough to provide a leaflet and perhaps a brief discussion with a healthcare professional.

The information given should be based on results from properly conducted scientific trials. Law[21] suggests that the scientific rigour which prevails in other areas of medicine may not always be applied to screening. He cites breast self-examination as one example of this. This has been widely advocated on the spurious assumption that it must be beneficial and cannot do harm. In fact it has been shown to be ineffective and to result in unnecessary surgical biopsies and considerable anxiety.

He stresses that giving information to people who are considering screening (e.g. on prostate-specific antigen (PSA) testing) when the only honest information available is complete uncertainty is useless, and that encouraging people to decide for themselves is evading the issue: 'For any cancer screening of unproved value it is unreasonable to expect that the investigation of screen positives or treatment of screen-detected cancers should be funded when healthcare resources are limited.'[21] He insists that the same rigour that is applied to the licensing of a new drug for general use should be applied to any new screening procedure.

Moynihan and colleagues[22] have drawn attention to the increasing problem of what they describe as 'disease-mongering' that often stems from pharmaceutical companies seeking to extend their markets: 'Disease-mongering can include turning ordinary ailments into medical problems, seeing mild symptoms as serious, treating personal problems as medical, seeing risks as disease, and framing prevalence estimates to maximise potential markets.'[22] Among other examples, they cite the transformation of baldness or shyness from ordinary processes of life into medical conditions amenable to treatment.

These authors suggest three steps to help redress the balance in this area.

1 Move away from using corporate-funded information on medical conditions/ diseases.
2 Generate independent, accessible material on conditions and diseases. Genuinely independent sources of information about health problems could replace those skewed towards making the maximum number of healthy people feel sick.
3 Widen notions of informed consent to include information about controversy surrounding the definition of conditions and diseases.

The public now has access to a great deal of information of variable respectability on health through the media and the Internet, and should theoretically be able to use this to assess the real value and possible risks of many tests and treatments. In reality, the situation is more complex and healthcare professionals need to be able to advise patients on where to find good-quality health information in a rapidly changing field.[23]

For example, in an analysis of 840 health news stories that appeared between February and May 2003 on four television stations in Minnesota, Schwitzer identified 10 troublesome trends in health reporting.[24] These included hyperbole such as the coverage of the use of Botox in pain control described by the single doctor who was interviewed as a 'miracle drug', creeping commercialism, and Food and Drug Administration (FDA) approval being regarded as a fait accompli for drugs still in the early stages of research.

A 1993 report from the Audit Commission found that many patients had experienced difficulties in obtaining relevant information about their conditions.[25] Consultation times can be too short for adequate explanation, healthcare professionals themselves may lack knowledge of treatment options and their likely effects, and the patient's wish or ability to cope with information may be underestimated.

In a review of patient information for 10 common conditions, Coulter and colleagues highlighted four specific issues that need to be addressed.[26]

• If information materials are to be used to support patients' involvement in treatment decisions, they must contain relevant, research-based data in a form that is acceptable and useful to patients.

- Current information materials for patients omit relevant data, fail to give a balanced view of the effectiveness of different treatments, and ignore uncertainties.
- Many information materials adopt a patronising tone, and few actively promote a participative approach to decision making.
- Groups that produce information materials must start with needs defined by patients, give treatment information that is based on rigorous systematic reviews, and involve multi-disciplinary teams (including patients) in developing and testing the materials.

These researchers called for various government measures to promote shared decision making based on the provision of good-quality information. These included ensuring that each NHS trust and primary care group have a designated senior member of staff responsible for ensuring that patient information meets high-quality standards, and that all clinicians receive training in communication skills and techniques.

Godolphin[27] argues for shared decision making as 'an ideal that aims to reconcile the fact of professional power with the ethic of informed choice.' Current medical training does not tend to foster the idea of offering choice or enhancing patient autonomy. He poses the question 'What would happen if "we have some choices and they are . . ." was in the doctor's habitual script, and "what's the evidence for that, doctor?" was in the patient's?'

In a systematic review of the use of decision aids for patients facing health treatment or screening decisions, O'Connor and colleagues[28] found that they improved knowledge, reduced conflict and helped patients to become more active in decision making without increasing their anxiety.

Barratt and colleagues[29] suggest that decision aids must include information about the whole screening process, including follow-up tests (some of which may be invasive and unpleasant) and treatments. The harms of screening are still poorly understood by the public, and screening tests are often viewed uncritically.

A recent report from the National Consumer Council[30] highlights the issue of health literacy defined as 'the capacity of an individual to obtain, interpret and understand basic health information and services in ways that are health-enhancing,' and calls for a more user-focused approach from the NHS in making information available in plain language, when and how patients from all groups want it.

Achieving truly informed consent through shared decision making in screening, as elsewhere in healthcare, is an admirable goal. It will take continued training and willingness to change the still prevalent attitude that 'doctor knows best' from healthcare professionals and patients alike to translate it into everyday practice.

Economic principles of screening

Economic aspects of screening have come to the fore in the consideration of screening in the last decade. This is partly because of theoretical advances in the application of economic principles in health services, but also because of the realisation that some screening procedures consume large amounts of money with little benefit to the population. Raffle has recently illustrated this by an analysis of the resources consumed in screening for cervical cancer and the number of curable cases identified.[31] With the increase in perception by both policy makers and the public that stringent criteria must be applied before screening procedures are introduced, economic facts have been increasingly demanded in order to try to quantify the costs and benefits in terms that are more readily understood.

As economic theory has entered the field, it has been increasingly recognised that screening is not a universal panacea and that it may also do harm. The topic thus joins the list of ethical considerations that need to be appreciated in any screening programme. As was discussed in Chapter 1, screening is a procedure that is used on populations in which large numbers of people are tested. Some of these individuals are likely to have apparently abnormal results and to require further testing to determine the validity of the findings. Those who are found to meet the set criteria can then be treated. However, as should be constantly reiterated, screening differs from normal medical practice in that the individuals who are undergoing a screening procedure are invited to participate with the implied promise that they will benefit. This contrasts with normal medical practice, where the patient approaches the medical practitioner with a symptom or complaint and requests help.

All screening procedures require the testing of large numbers of individuals in order to find the few with an abnormality. There are two main consequences of this.

First, those who undergo screening are often understandably anxious while waiting for the result, and become even more anxious if they have to undergo further investigation.[32] These further investigations may not be pain or risk free (e.g. amniocentesis for Down's syndrome causes abortion in about 1% of those who undergo it), and thus may induce 'illness' in those who previously considered themselves to be well. Increasingly, people who are found to be normal still have a residual anxiety that something may be wrong.

Secondly, population-screening procedures involve the examination and testing of large numbers of people in order to detect a few abnormalities. Although most screening tests are simple and relatively cheap procedures in themselves, the actual costs are by no means trivial because of the large numbers involved. Some screening tests that are advocated (often by 'for-profit' providers), such as whole body scanning,[33] are expensive. Further investigation of those found to be positive on screening, many of whom will eventually prove to be negative, is also likely to be expensive. Since the amount of resources available for health services is constrained, it is essential that the costs of screening services are considered when evaluating whether such services are justified in competition with other services, such as better caring services for the elderly and chronic sick, or services for another patient group.

In the application of economic methods, economists develop econometric models whereby the economic consequences of activities are estimated. In developing models for cancer screening, Mansley and McKenna[34] considered it important to develop specific models from a variety of different perspectives. For example, the model constructed from the viewpoint of an individual patient will be mainly concerned with the decisions made for that patient by the healthcare professionals, whether a screening test is positive or negative. The family's perspective will be largely concerned with the health outcomes of the findings.

The employer's perspective will focus on secondary and non-health outcomes. Mansley and McKenna identified eight perspectives and then tried to determine which component was economically most important. They illustrated the application of these principles to cancer screening, and demonstrated that for most areas and conditions there are few facts available and this limits the potential for and usefulness of econometric approaches.

In fiscal terms, they estimated the costs in the USA of follow-up diagnostic procedures to screening mammography (diagnostic X-ray, ultrasound, fine-needle aspiration, biopsy, repeat examinations or surgical consultations), and concluded that the cost of these 1818 procedures per 10 000 mammograms is about US$235 000.

Sassi[35] goes further in considering the need for an economic evaluation of the diagnostic process in screening.

The first stage of an economic evaluation requires examination of the production of the test result – that is, the sensitivity and specificity in relation to the population tested. The second stage involves the use of the diagnostic output of screening as part of a diagnostic strategy and choice of treatment 'which entails the estimation of post-test probabilities of disease using a Bayesian rule and the choice of treatment on the basis of disease probability thresholds balancing alternative possible outcomes.'[35] The third stage of the evaluation is the production of final outcomes conditional upon the choice of treatment. He illustrates the complexity of the required evaluation and suggests possible solutions.

The health outcome of a screening test may produce true as well as false results. As we have already stated, the result of a screening test may produce a health effect (e.g. increased sickness absence by individuals labelled as positive) and the test itself may have a short-term effect (e.g. pain). These factors all have to be considered in economic terms of costs and benefits. The reassurance or distress of the individual undergoing screening thus has economic as well as psychological or behavioural consequences, although these are not usually measured or known.

The clinician's behaviour is also affected by the possible need to undertake further diagnostic tests to help give reassurance either for not providing treatment or for starting the necessary therapy.

Psychological variables need to be taken into account in the development of an economic evaluative model. These would include the likelihood of a patient's or clinician's willingness to take risks, the empathy and emotional relationship between the clinician and the patient, which may have a bearing on the actions undertaken, and, above all, limitations in our knowledge of the consequences of the tests or treatments and the behavioural/attitudinal/psychological implications for the patient.

In an econometric model, the question of incentives for specific actions needs to be taken into account. Thus in medical screening the practitioner may order specific tests that enhance or diminish the fees paid. There may also be non-financial incentives for specific tests or actions, such as the need to be able to demonstrate to peers and patients the clinician's expertise and familiarity with technological possibilities.

Sassi continues by outlining the major problems, such as opportunity costs, particularly when shared resources are involved. One example of this, that has already been mentioned, was in the early days of cervical cytology when smears were examined by pathologists rather than by laboratory technicians. This increased workload resulted in the performance of fewer post-mortem examinations.

Most workers implicitly but wrongly assume that when a test is introduced, capacity is increased (e.g. by the employment of extra staff, or by the purchase of new machinery). Even if this was the case, and often it is not, as the example above illustrates, the costs of advertising, hiring and accommodating new staff and providing additional space for new machinery all have to be taken into account.

The complexity of economic evaluation is well illustrated by Sassi's consideration of some of the factors that impact on diagnostic decisions. These are summarised in Table 2.1.

For the development of adequate methods of costing screening services, where shared resources are employed in the production process, most workers have used methods which may not be able to provide adequate estimates of opportunity costs. Sassi states that information is needed not only on the individuals undergoing testing but also on the costs and benefits to other patients or individuals who would, or would not, have access to the test(s), as a consequence of decisions regarding the use of those test(s). Furthermore, when deciding whether to introduce a new test, the global cost-effectiveness of shared resources should be evaluated rather than the cost-effectiveness of the individual test alone. Thus evaluations require the determination of what case mix would allow a satisfactory absorption of fixed costs, given the cost-effectiveness of using shares of production capacity for specific groups of patients, before allocating the cost of shared resources.

Sassi conducted a cost-effectiveness analysis of cervical cancer screening based on:

> a cross-sectional mathematical model comparing the current strategy to the one in use prior to the introduction of target payments, and to possible alternative strategies that may further improve the effectiveness of the programme. With the introduction of target payments 259

Table 2.1 Complexity of economic evaluation: factors and impact

Factor	Impact
Health outcomes	True results (positive and negative) False results (positive and negative) 'Psychologically mediated' health effects Short-term health outcomes
Reassurance and distress	For the patient (e.g. prenatal screening, screening for breast cancer) For the clinician (e.g. ordering of laboratory tests)
Psychological variables	Cognitive response style (risk aversion) – patient Cognitive response style (risk aversion) – clinician Emotional response style (sympathy/empathy) Cognitive limitations
Incentives	Financial (e.g. response to changes in relative fees) Non-financial (technological imperative)

cancer deaths are avoided and 4045 life-years are gained every year at a cost-effectiveness ratio of £13 957 per life-year gained. Further improvements may be obtained by increasing coverage among groups with a lower uptake, such as women in disadvantaged socio-economic conditions or from ethnic minorities, at a cost-effectiveness ratio of £22 073 per life-year gained, or by shortening screening interval, at a cost-effectiveness ratio of £14 808 per life-year gained. Despite high cost, the current programme produced significant benefits.[35]

Using this model, Sassi suggests that there is scope for further improvements by increasing coverage while maintaining a three- or five-year interval. However, this would entail an increase in NHS expenditure that might not be feasible.

Sassi and colleagues,[36] using these approaches, have raised the issue of equity versus efficiency. In cervical cancer screening, the policy aim is to maximise coverage by economic incentives to general practices. However, less affluent women in England have a lower participation rate in this programme than their more affluent counterparts. Equivalent cost-effectiveness ratios for cervical cancer screening could be achieved with less frequent but more even coverage. This is, of course, particularly important in a condition such as cervical cancer which is more common among more deprived women.

Another example where such mathematical–economic models are helpful is in the formulation of policy for sickle-cell disease screening. This condition particularly affects certain ethnic-minority groups. Current recommendations (*see* Chapter 4) advocate the use of universal screening when the relevant ethnic-minority groups account for 15% of the population or more. The cost of this is £430 000 to £1 million per life-year saved compared with selective screening, the variation being attributable to the proportion of high-risk births. This is more effective but more expensive than selective screening. However, the choice between universal and selective screening may have important distributional implications. Universal screening does not seem to be justified, as there is no benefit of this policy for white European babies. Thus significant efficiency gains may be sacrificed for what seems to be an inappropriate concept of equity.

This brief description of some of the economic considerations used in the evaluation of screening procedures demonstrates the complexity of the problem, the need to develop appropriate economic models and perspectives and the need to avoid the somewhat simplistic methods that are still commonly used. Finally, as Mushin and colleagues assert, cost-effectiveness analyses require clinical information as well as economic data:

> Physicians and medical scientists should therefore participate to make the conclusions more scientifically robust and clinically valid. Although these analyses are designed to inform government or medical system decision makers, they provide clinicians with information that will be essential in their roles as medical practitioners and, perhaps most importantly, as responsible advocates for the best healthcare possible.[37]

Conclusion

The key issues of genetics, information and economics discussed in this chapter are impossible to separate sensibly from ethics and audit, which form the substance of Chapter 3. All of these overlapping elements must be at the forefront of any discussion of screening.

Genetic screening has developed very rapidly and although it has huge potential, caution and sensitivity in its use are paramount. Its main purpose at present is to prevent rather than treat disease. In this it differs from much of current screening practice, and it must not be allowed to overlook the basic principles and criteria of screening. Open debate on the best way forward is urgently needed, and the ethical and human implications of the use of the human genome must be considered and patient autonomy guarded.

Information is another central concept in modern healthcare in general and screening in particular. Information must be provided not, as has so often been the case in the past, with the purpose of encouraging participation in a programme, but rather to give a balanced and understandable picture of the options and the possible outcomes with the endpoint of truly informed consent.

A screening service that is provided for one population consumes resources which will not then be available for use elsewhere. Economic approaches may demonstrate conflicting aspects of policy decisions. For example, increasing efficiency may reduce equity. They may also highlight the differing perspectives of providers, consumers and industry. In a health service where financial resources are and will continue to be insufficient, expert economic analysis and advice must be an integral part of the system and must help to guide policy.

References

1 Holtzman NA and Watson MS (eds) (1999) *Promoting Safe and Effective Genetic Testing. Final Report of the Task Force on Genetic Testing.* Johns Hopkins University Press, Baltimore, MD.
2 Burke W (2002) Genetic testing. *NEJM.* **347**: 1867–75.
3 www.geneclinics.org
4 Burgermeister J (2003) Teacher was refused job because relatives have Huntington's disease (news item). *BMJ.* **327**: 827.
5 Stone DH and Stewart S (1996) Screening and the new genetics: a public health perspective on the ethical debate. *J Public Health Med.* **18**: 3–5.
6 Ridley M (1999) *Genome.* Fourth Estate, London.
7 Pinsky LE *et al.* (2001) Genetic testing for breast and ovarian cancer susceptibility: a public health perspective. *West Med J.* **175**: 168–73.
8 www.cdc.gov/genomics/info/perspectives/breastcancer.htm
9 Colhoun HM, McKeigue PM and Davey Smith G (2003) Problems of reporting genetic associations with complex outcomes. *Lancet.* **361**: 865–72.
10 Broadstock M, Michie S and Marteau T (2000) Psychological consequences of predictive genetic testing: a systematic review. *Eur J Hum Genet.* **8**: 731–8.
11 Harper PS, Lim C and Crauford D on behalf of the UK Huntington's Disease Prediction Consortium (2000) Ten years of presymptomatic testing for Huntington's disease: the experience of the UK Huntington's Disease Prediction Consortium. *J Med Genet.* **37**: 567–71.

12 Binidell J, Soldan JR and Harper PS (1998) Predictive testing for Huntington's disease. II. Qualitative findings from a study of uptake in South Wales. *Clin Genet.* **54**: 489–96.

13 Melzer D and Zimmern R (2002) Genetics and medicalisation (editorial). *BMJ.* **324**: 863–4.

14 Holtzman NA (1996) Medical and ethical issues in genetic screening – an academic view. *Environ Health Perspect.* **104 (Suppl. 5)**: 987–90.

15 Burke W, Coughlin SS, Lee NC, Weed DL and Khoury MJ (2001) Application of population screening principles to genetic screening for adult-onset conditions. *Genet Test.* **5**: 201–11.

16 Anderlik MR and Rothstein DA (2004) Privacy and confidentiality of genetic information – what rules for the new science? *Annu Rev Genomics Hum Genet.* **2**: 401–33.

17 Parens E and Asch A (2003) Disability rights critique of prenatal genetic testing: reflections and recommendations. *Ment Retard Dev Disabil Res Rev.* **1**: 40–47.

18 Vineis P, Schulte P and McMichael AJ (2001) Misconceptions about the use of genetic tests in populations. *Lancet.* **357**: 709–12.

19 Samavat A and Modell B (2004) Iranian national thalassaemia screening programme. *BMJ.* **329**: 1134–7.

20 Tryggvadøttir L (2000) Cancer registries and genetic screening. In: *European Commission on Europe against Cancer Programme, IARC, European Network of Cancer Registries.* European Commission, Brussels.

21 Law M (2004) Screening without evidence of efficacy (editorial). *BMJ.* **328**: 301–2.

22 Moynihan R, Heath I and Henry DE (2002) Selling sickness: the pharmaceutical industry and disease mongering. *BMJ.* **324**: 886–91.

23 Shepperd S, Charnock D and Gann B (1999) Helping patients access high-quality health information. *BMJ.* **319**: 764–6.

24 Schwitzer G (2004) Ten troublesome trends in TV health news. *BMJ.* **329**: 1352.

25 Audit Commission (1993) *What Seems to be the Matter: communication between hospitals and patients.* HMSO, London.

26 Coulter A, Entwistle V and Gilbert D (1999) Sharing decisions with patients: is the information good enough? *BMJ.* **318**: 318–22.

27 Godolphin W (2003) The role of risk communication in shared decision making (editorial). *BMJ.* **327**: 692–3.

28 O'Connor A, Rostom A, Fiset V *et al.* (1999) Decision aids for patients facing health treatments or screening decisions: systematic review. *BMJ.* **319**: 731–4.

29 Barratt A, Trevena L, Davey HM and McCaffery K (2004) Use of decision aids to support informed choices about screening. *BMJ.* **329**: 507–10.

30 Sihota S and Lennard L (2004) *Health Literacy.* National Consumer Council, London.

31 Raffle AE, Alden B, Quinn M, Babb J and Brett MT (2003) Outcomes of screening to prevent cancer: analysis of cumulative incidence of cervical abnormality and modelling of cases and deaths prevented. *BMJ.* **326**: 901–9.

32 Marteau TM, Cook R, Kidd J *et al.* (1992) The psychological effects of false-positive results in prenatal screening for fetal abnormalities: a prospective study. *Prenat Diagn.* **12**: 205–14.

33 Smith R (2003) The screening industry (editorial). *BMJ.* **326**: 891.

34 Mansley EC and McKenna MT (2001) Importance of perspective in economic analyses of cancer screening decisions. *Lancet.* **358**: 1169–73.

35 Sassi F (2000) *The outcomes of medical diagnosis on economic perspective.* PhD thesis, London. London School of Economics and London University.

36 Sassi F, Le Grand J and Archard L (2001) Equity versus efficiency: a dilemma for the NHS. *BMJ.* **323**: 762–3.

37 Mushin AI, Rushlin HS and Callahan MA (2001) Cost-effectiveness of diagnostic tests. *Lancet.* **358**: 1353–5.

Chapter 3

Key issues in screening: ethics and audit

Disease has many faces and the hunt is not benign.*

Introduction

Two aspects of screening, namely ethics and audit or quality control, form the substance of this chapter and are of the utmost importance. Ethical consider-ations, such as the harm-to-benefit ratio, must be paramount whenever a screening programme is considered for implementation. In the same way, audit, evaluation and quality control are essential elements without which screening is at best useless and at worst immoral.

Ethics of screening

As we have stated earlier, screening differs significantly from normal medical practice. In traditional medical practice individuals seek help from a doctor because they have symptoms and want to be reassured or diagnosed and treated appropriately. In population screening, on the other hand, the health service invites individuals who consider themselves to be well to undergo an examina-tion or to be tested in order that a particular condition can be identified at an early stage so that treatment may be given while the condition is reversible or at least containable. The situation is thus crucially different in that the service and not the individual has initiated the contact. Those who undergo screening examinations cannot therefore be considered as patients, although they may of course *become* patients who require treatment as a result of screening.

The question of opportunistic screening in primary care is rather different but no less difficult ethically. A patient may present at surgery with a health problem, and the general practitioner may take the opportunity to suggest various other tests, such as the measurement of blood pressure or cholesterol, appropriate to the individual's age and sex.

Getz and colleagues are among those who are now questioning the legitimacy of this: 'Most medical experts and health authorities consider consultations in primary health care ideal for opportunistic health promotion and disease pre-vention. Doctors are thus expected to discuss preventive measures even when they are not among the reasons for contact.'[1] They question whether such initiatives are ethically justifiable in contemporary Western medicine, and

* Berwick DM (1985) Scoliosis screening: a pause in the chase. *Am J Public Health.* **75**: 1373–4.

argue that doctors should 'maintain a clear focus on each patient's reasons for seeking help rather than be distracted by an increasing list of standardised preventive measures with unpredictable relevance to the individual.'

This thinking had its roots almost 30 years ago when Ivan Illich published his then controversial critique of modern medicine in which he voiced the view that 'modern medicine has become a major threat to health.'[2] He contended that medicine had destroyed the ability of people to cope with difficulties that are part of everyday life, preferring instead the illusion that death, pain and sickness can be defeated. Illich did not suggest the dismantling of medicine, but advocated 'sanitation, inoculation and vector control, well-distributed health education, healthy architecture, and safe machinery, general competence in first aid, equally distributed access to dental and primary medical care, as well as judiciously selected complex services.'[2] How sensible this sounds now to those who are in favour of de-medicalisation and increased patient power – but how heretical it seemed in 1976.

As Moynihan and Smith[3] have pointed out, there is a move now to shift power from doctors to patients, to encourage autonomy and self-care and to resist attempts to medicalise life problems such as shyness, loneliness or ageing. The growth of the Internet, providing information – be it correct or spurious – on health and disease, enables individuals to be much better informed about their health. This is no longer a radical agenda.

The ethical perspective is thus very different. In screening, any abnormalities that are identified must be treatable and the investigation itself must not do any harm. Cochrane and Holland[4] compared the situation to that of the salesman who stands up in the marketplace and tries to sell a cough medicine – there will be no buyers unless the cough medicine is shown to suppress coughing.

As a result of this difference a number of principles need to be fulfilled before screening procedures are advocated or introduced into practice as outlined in Chapter 1. The most crucial criterion is that an effective method of treatment is available for those identified by screening as abnormal. Implicit in this is that individuals move from considering themselves to be well to having a condition or an abnormality, and that this change occurs at a time when the likelihood of effective treatment and survival is enhanced.

However, there are a number of additional issues that require consideration. All studies of screening have been conducted on defined population groups (e.g. the inhabitants of a town or the children in a school). In such situations, the number of individuals found to have a positive test result is likely to be small, but the benefit is assessed in terms of the improvement in health (survival) of the population investigated. This illustrates Rose's preventive paradox, in which a preventive measure can bring much benefit to a population but offers little to each participating individual.[5]

In all instances there are going to be disadvantages to some members of the population screened. All screening examinations are preliminary and will entail further investigation to verify that those who screen positive really do have the abnormality and require treatment (*true positives*), and to eliminate those who screen positive but do not actually have the abnormality (*false positives*). Those individuals with negative test results will not normally be tested further, although some of them may actually have the abnormality in question (*false negatives*). This obviously has serious implications, as will be discussed below.

There remains confusion among both the public and the health professions with regard to the use of the various terms surrounding screening, and thus the ethical considerations. The main confusion is between the concepts of 'individual good' and 'community good.' Any individuals who are identified as having a treatable condition at an early stage and are receiving effective treatment will consider themselves to be fortunate, and may find it difficult to understand why screening policies are not advocated universally for 'their' condition. The difficulty in discussions on screening and the reason why stringent principles must be followed is that screening may also cause harm.

Since a screening test is performed on a large number of people, it is inevitable that there will be some individuals in the population tested who are false negatives as mentioned above – that is, they show a negative result but actually have the condition in question. These individuals will be reassured falsely that they are healthy. Screening tests, even with all the safeguards, can never be foolproof and are subject to human and technical error and variation, so that even with the most thorough quality assurance mechanisms, mistakes will occur. In any assessment of screening in a population an assessment has to be made of the harm–benefit ratio.

A further difficulty arises in the ethical evaluation of screening. There must always be a time interval between conducting a screening test, receiving the result, performing the diagnostic test and receiving that result. Numerous studies (e.g. those by Austoker[6] and Marteau and colleagues[7]) have shown that in some cases considerable anxiety develops in those who have been tested, both in those found to be negative and those who eventually receive treatment. This anxiety must be taken into account when the introduction of any screening test is being considered.

The semantics of screening are also important. We have described both population and opportunistic screening. In colloquial language, however, the situation can also arise where an individual goes to a doctor to request a specific test to determine whether he or she is suffering from a particular condition. The ethical situation in this case is very different from that in population or even opportunistic screening – as the individual has initiated the request for screening, not the doctor.

Account must also be taken of screening performed as a protective measure to identify an illness or condition in individuals, not necessarily for treatment but to prevent others from coming into contact with them and becoming ill or infected.

Two examples of this are tuberculosis and severe acute respiratory syndrome (SARS). This is a difficult area ethically, since one of the main criteria for screening, namely the availability of effective treatment or management, may not be able to be fulfilled.

In the case of tuberculosis, mass X-ray screening was used not only to identify people with early disease so that they could be treated, but also to provide information and advice about avoiding contact with those individuals, such as children and the elderly, who might be especially susceptible.

More controversially, it has recently been suggested that individuals with early signs of SARS, such as high fever, should be identified and kept in isolation in order to prevent the spread of the infection, for which there is currently no effective treatment.

The public perception of screening – often encouraged by the media – tends to be positive despite these complex ethical considerations. Many believe that early diagnosis, particularly of cancer and heart disease, will lead to the possibility of treatment and improvement in prognosis. This is an attractive concept and can lead to a demand for screening procedures to be introduced irrespective of whether it has been shown that diagnosis guarantees an improved outcome. The belief that identifying the presence of a condition equates with the ability to alter its natural history may beguile the public, but is unfortunately false.

Commercial interests can also be involved. Many industries now provide materials, equipment and even screening facilities. Health checks are now being advertised by private healthcare providers, and whole body scanning is being promoted, especially in the USA, with the frightening prospect of abnormalities being found without consideration of any of the basic principles of screening or its possible harmful effects. Nor is advocacy of screening limited to particular industries that produce the particular machinery or reagents. It is encouraged by insurers and private healthcare providers who may wish to use the results not only for the benefit (or otherwise) of the individual, but also to identify people who might not be a 'good risk.'

Demand for screening services is also promoted by individual charities that are concerned with the well-being of one particular patient group. The recent experience of Professor Alan Coates, Head of the Cancer Council Australia, with regard to screening for prostate cancer provides a stark example of the danger of excessive advocacy.

Professor Coates stated openly that he would not undergo a prostate-specific antigen (PSA) test for prostate cancer because there was insufficient evidence of benefit, and the invasive follow-up procedures to an abnormal test result might outweigh any advantage. He was subsequently subjected to a barrage of letters, emails and press articles from politicians, urologists, other medical practitioners and members of the public, all critical of his stance. The attacks were orchestrated by the Australian Prostate Cancer Foundation, which is supported by an unnamed financial services company whose propaganda is co-ordinated without charge by a large advertising agency.

In another episode of the bullying tactics of the pro-screening lobby for this condition, an article published in the *Western Medical Journal* in the USA which questioned the wisdom of PSA testing at this time was viciously attacked by the local prostate cancer charities.

Commenting on the PSA testing furore in the *Sydney Morning Herald*,[8] Chapman pointed out that although mortality from prostate cancer in Australia has increased in the past decade, mortality in the only randomised controlled trial of screening for the condition was similar in the screening and non-screening groups: 'Simply finding cancer is never the goal of screening.'

The ethics of screening is an immensely complex subject and does require further debate and clarification in view of ever advancing technology. As was mentioned in the previous chapter, Stone and Stewart[9] assert that information gathered, for example, in the course of genetic carrier screening cannot be assumed to be of benefit merely by asserting a 'right to know' imperative. We must also accept the right of individuals *not* to know, and be constantly mindful of long-established screening principles.

The issue of patient autonomy deserves to be revisited in the light of the rapid expansion of preventive medicine.[10] Patient autonomy includes 'a person's freedom to consider, choose or reject preventive or therapeutic options after receiving sufficient information.'[11] However, information about medical risk once imparted cannot be retracted: 'Respect for autonomy should therefore also honour the person's right not to be opportunistically confronted with knowledge about biomedical risks that are unrelated to his or her reasons for seeing the doctor.'[12]

Audit, evaluation and quality control

In any screening programme, as with any other service programme, adequate steps must be taken to ensure that the original objectives are being met and that the methodology meets appropriate standards.

The general objective of screening is to reduce mortality and morbidity – that is, to identify a condition at a stage when it is reversible or at least containable. The various criteria that need to be satisfied have been described in Chapter 1.

The ideal method for evaluating a screening programme is the randomised controlled trial, in which individuals in a population are allocated at random either to a group that is screened or to a group that receives only its normal medical care. The South-East London Multiphasic Screening Study (SELSS), which reported in 1977, was an example of such a trial.[13] In this study all adults aged 40–64 years on the lists of two large group practices were allocated at random by family to either of two groups, one group receiving screening and the other receiving their normal medical care. The screening group was re-screened after two years and both groups were then examined four years after the initial randomisation. The end points are shown in Table 3.1.

This design enabled the investigators to avoid some of the common biases that bedevil the evaluation of screening.

The first of these is *lead-time bias*. Lead-time is the interval between the time of detection of a condition by screening and the time at which it would have been diagnosed in the absence of screening.

The second bias is *length-biased sampling*. Individuals who have rapidly progressing disease will tend to develop symptoms that cause them to consult a GP immediately, and thus only less rapidly progressive cases are likely to be detected

Table 3.1 Summary of end points in the South-East London Multiphasic Screening Study[13]

End point	Measures
Mortality	Death from all causes and from specific diseases such as coronary heart disease and cancer
Morbidity	Sickness absence for the employed Use of home helps for women not in employment Use of clinical services (e.g. clinical services, general practitioners)
Levels of function	Blood pressure Breathlessness Mobility

by screening. The former, of course, have a poorer prognosis than the latter, and therefore the results will tend to suggest that screening is more effective than is really the case.

The third bias is *selection bias*. Since any participant in a screening study is a volunteer, it is likely that those who are most health-conscious will participate, and they are likely to survive longer in any case, whether they are screened or not. In the SELSS, for example, about 70% of the population who were invited participated. Those who refused had a higher mortality in the first year compared with the participants.

Fourthly, *over-diagnosis bias* means that some of the lesions that are identified, which are counted as disease, may not present clinically during their lifetime. This is one of the probable reasons for the excess of prostate cancer identified by the PSA test compared with the mortality from prostate cancer.

Randomised controlled trials are expensive and difficult to manage, and may also be ethically unacceptable, as experience with screening for cervical cancer suggests. A national cervical cancer screening programme was established in the UK in 1964 without sufficient evidence that the identification of an abnormal smear with the possibility of further investigation and treatment would reduce mortality from the condition. By the time that serious doubts about the effectiveness and organisation of the programme began to be raised, a randomised controlled trial was ethically impossible, since women would not have wanted to be included in the control group. Comparisons have been made of the mortality rates for women due to cancer of the cervix in areas where the service has been well organised and where the uptake has been good, compared with areas where the service has been less well organised and controlled. Time trends have been examined, and these suggest that screening for cervical cancer is effective in reducing mortality.

Finally, a number of services have been evaluated on the basis of case–control studies by comparing the screening history of individuals with the condition sought with the screening history of individuals from a comparable population who do not have the disease. Of course these studies are subject to all the disadvantages of case–control studies.

In view of all these potential problems, the National Screening Committee only recommends the introduction of any new screening programme after assessment of the findings of a properly conducted randomised controlled trial. It is also essential that all screening programmes are kept under regular scrutiny to ensure that they continue to perform in the way intended and continue to be effective.

The components of an effectively organised screening programme have been summarised by Hakama.[14] We have modified these to the following.

1   Identification of the target population.
2   Identification of the individuals in the population to be screened.
3   Means to ensure that all those eligible for screening can attend (e.g. a personal invitation, suitable timing of screening examinations to suit the needs of those involved).
4   Adequate premises, equipment and staff to ensure that the screening examination is conducted under pleasant conditions and is acceptable to those attending.

5   An appropriate, satisfactory method of ensuring the maintenance of the best standards of the test(s) – that is, quality assurance by:
    *   initial and continuing training of the personnel conducting the test(s)
    *   demonstration (by appropriate records) of the maintenance standards of equipment used in the examination (e.g. calibration of X-ray machines in mammography)
    *   routine checks of the validity of the tests performed (e.g. random duplicate measurements for biochemistry, cytology, and reading of X-rays).

6   Adequate and appropriate facilities for the diagnosis and treatment of any individual found to require this. There should be as little delay as possible between the screening attendance, advice that the screening test was negative, advice that the screening test result required further investigation, and referral to the appropriate centre for further investigation or treatment. A timetable should be established for these different procedures, and there should be continuous monitoring to ensure that the time intervals between the various stages are complied with.

7   There should be regular checks on the feelings of satisfaction of those who have undergone the screening process – including those investigated, the screen-negatives and those who were invited who have not participated.

8   Finally, regular periodic checks should be made of the records of the screened individuals to ascertain their adequacy.

The importance of maintaining the quality of screening programmes should never be underestimated. The regular scare stories in the media of failures in the cervical cancer and breast cancer screening programmes could largely be avoided by stringent quality control, although some error is inevitable. Sasieni and Cuzick have proposed that routine audit should be an ethical requirement of any screening programme,[15] and that there should be regulations in accordance with clause 68 of the Health and Social Care Bill to ensure this.

The problems of ensuring the quality of even the technical parts of screening should not be underestimated. Smith, for example, has raised the question of the accuracy and variability of results of genetic screening.[16] Furthermore, attention has recently been drawn to the possibility of interference in immunoassays, which is difficult to detect and could affect patient care adversely. Such interference is specific to each individual, so only that individual's data will be affected and quality assurance criteria for the assay will not have been met. Inaccurate reporting of endocervical components of Pap smears still occurs and can result in slide re-screens, amended reports, clinician dissatisfaction and sometimes unnecessary repeat screens.[17] Difficulties with regard to the verification of the quality and safety of health information services, with the increasing use of clinical software, telemedicine and the Internet, have also been reported.[18]

As Miller has stated in his discussion of the prerequisites for successful screening programmes, quality assurance is much more than quality assurance in laboratories:[19] 'An effective organised programme is one that is adequately planned, on the basis of the needs and resources of a country or region, one that is adequately funded and one that is efficiently managed.' Only by a continuous programme of education, training and rigorous adherence to sound protocols and principles can screening meet its objectives. Quality must exist throughout the screening pathway.

Conclusion

Ethics and audit are both in different ways fundamental to the integrity of any screening programme.

Through advances in technology, the potential for testing – particularly in the field of genetics – is immense. More than ever before it is vital that the basic principles on which screening should be based remain in sharp focus. The technical ability to perform a screening procedure does not guarantee its ethical acceptability, as many experiments in other areas of science and medicine currently illustrate. The criteria for screening, first promulgated by Wilson and Jungner,[20] and described in Chapter 1, must be satisfied before any screening test or programme can be considered ethical.

In line with this, audit and quality control should be an integral part of screening to ensure that it is achieving what it has set out to do in a way that is acceptable to those involved.

References

1 Getz L, Sigurdsson JA and Hetlevik I (2003) Is opportunistic disease prevention in the consultation ethically justifiable? *BMJ.* **327**: 498–500.
2 Illich I (1976) *Limits to Medicine*. Marion Boyars, London.
3 Moynihan R and Smith R (2002) Too much medicine? (editorial). *BMJ.* **324**: 859–60.
4 Cochrane AL and Holland WW (1971) Validation of screening procedures. *Br Med Bull.* **27**: 3–8.
5 Rose G (1985) Sick individuals and sick populations. *Int J Epidemiol.* **14**: 32–8.
6 Austoker J (1999) Gaining informed consent for screening (editorial). *BMJ.* **319**: 722–3.
7 Marteau TM, Kidd J, Michie S, Cook R, Johnston M and Shaw RW (1993) Anxiety, knowledge and satisfaction in women receiving false-positive results on routine prenatal screening: a randomised controlled trial. *J Psychometr Obstet Gynaecol.* **14**: 185–96.
8 Chapman S (2003) Fresh rows over prostate screening. *BMJ.* **326**: 605.
9 Stone DH and Stewart S (1996) Screening and the new genetics: a public health perspective on the ethical debate. *J Public Health Med.* **18**: 3–5.
10 Getz L and Kirkengen AL (2003) Ultrasound screening in pregnancy: advancing technology, soft markers for fetal chromosomal aberrations, and unacknowledged ethical dilemmas. *Soc Sci Med.* **56**: 2045–57.
11 Tauber AI (2001) Historical and philosophical reflections on patient autonomy. *Health Care Anal.* **9**: 299–319.
12 Getz L, Nilsson PM and Hetlevik I (2003) A matter of heart: the general practitioner consultation in an evidence-based world. *Scand J Prim Health Care.* **21**: 3–9.
13 South-East London Screening Study Group (1977) A controlled trial of multiphasic screening in middle age. *Int J Epidemiol.* **6**: 357–63.
14 Hakama M (1986) Screening for cancer. *Scand J Soc Med Suppl.* **37**: 17–25.
15 Sasieni P and Cuzick J (2001) Routine audit is an ethical requirement of screening. *BMJ.* **322**: 1179–80.
16 Smith KC (1998) Equivocal notions of accuracy and genetic screening of the general population. *Mt Sinai J Med.* **65**: 178–84.
17 Robertson J, Connolly K, St John K, Eltoum I and Chhieng DC (2002) Accuracy of reporting endocervical component adequacy – a continuous quality improvement project. *Diagn Cytopathol.* **27**: 181–4.
18 Rigby M, Forsstrom J, Roberts R and Wyatt J (2001) Verifying quality and safety in health informatics services. *BMJ.* **322**: 552–6.

19 Miller AB (2002) Quality assurance in screening strategies. *Virus Res.* **89**: 295–9.
20 Wilson JMG and Jungner G (1968) *Principles and Practice of Screening for Disease.* World Health Organization, Geneva.

Chapter 4

Antenatal and neonatal screening

> The provision of screening in general, including antenatal and neonatal screening, needs to be co-ordinated within a responsible public health screening service so that all screening programmes are well chosen, effectively implemented and continually researched. This is the greatest challenge in antenatal and neonatal screening.*

Introduction

In his foreword to the second edition of *Antenatal and Neonatal Screening*,[1] Sir Richard Doll drew attention to the demographic changes in developed countries, where birth rates continue to fall and life expectancy continues to rise: 'In these circumstances it is more than ever important that every newborn child should be both wanted and able to enjoy a full life unhampered by physical or mental disability.'

He also pointed out that developments in molecular biology have increased the number of situations in which intervention might be productive, but cautions that the possibility of effective intervention is not in itself an adequate reason for screening. At this stage of the life cycle, as at any other, it is vital to ensure that the long-established criteria for screening, described in Chapter 1, are met before screening is contemplated.

The aim of the National Screening Committee is to produce a single co-ordinated Antenatal and Neonatal Screening Programme, but here we shall consider screening under the separate antenatal and neonatal headings that best describe immediate reality.

Antenatal screening

What we are concerned with in this chapter, as throughout the book, is screening of the population to identify conditions in which more benefit than harm will result from early identification. This is perhaps particularly relevant in the antenatal period, which for the majority of pregnant women is a happy and productive period that we should not seek to medicalise.

We shall begin with an overview of current practice in antenatal screening in the UK, and then consider candidates for routine screening – with particular reference to the use of ultrasound and screening for Down's syndrome.

Antenatal care has been part of general practice for many years, and has often been quoted as an example of effective prevention at work. For example, in 1980 the Short Committee on Maternity Services stated: 'We unhesitatingly accept the

---

* Wald and Leck.[6]

often reiterated claim of antenatal care as a means of reducing perinatal and neonatal mortality.'[2]

Twelve years later, Jewell stated that it was becoming difficult to justify continuing the long-established practice of antenatal care in its traditional form, since health in general had improved and rates of maternal, fetal and neonatal mortality had declined.[3]

His view was that the key to good antenatal practice was the thorough application of effective screening tests (e.g. for bacteriuria, rubella and syphilis) early in pregnancy to prevent avoidable morbidity. Encouraging women to give up smoking and limit their consumption of alcohol would also improve outcome. He doubted the sense of the 'universal application of high-technology techniques, of doubtful value, to all pregnant women in the quest for perfect outcomes.' However, he warned that the benefits to women of regular attendance at antenatal clinics in terms of their emotional and psychological well-being, and to healthcare professionals in increasing their knowledge of individual patients, were also important and should not be overlooked. The ability to forestall hazards to the mother's health, such as pre-eclampsia, should also not be forgotten.

The two main sources of official advice on antenatal screening in the UK are the National Institute for Clinical Excellence (NICE)[4] and the UK National Screening Committee (NSC) and its Antenatal Screening Subgroup (ANSG).[5] In addition, Wald and Leck, in the second edition of *Antenatal and Neonatal Screening*,[6] have brought together the views of many specialists in this area.

The recommendations that these sources make vary according to their stance. NICE provides a simple and sensible guide to practice in routine antenatal care. The NSC, on advice from the ANSG, provides policy guidance to the Government, and its recommendations are hedged around with reviews and research. Wald and Leck and their contributors from their academic viewpoint recommend many more conditions for screening which may not be practicable in the real world of finite resources in terms of manpower and money.

In 2003, NICE published its guidelines on antenatal care.[4] These emphasised the importance of providing evidence-based information to enable women and their partners to make informed decisions about their antenatal care. The schedule of appointments should also be appropriate to the individual woman. Ten appointments should be adequate for a woman in a first uncomplicated pregnancy. For a subsequent uncomplicated pregnancy, seven appointments should suffice.

The NICE recommendations on antenatal screening, summarised in Table 4.1, provide a sensible framework for practice in the normal care of pregnant women.

The basis for the NSC's advice on antenatal as on all other stages of screening is evidence from randomised controlled trials or systematic reviews of controlled trials. However, the Committee and its Antenatal Subgroup also have to be sure that an equal standard of professional performance can be successfully transported from the research setting into national practice.

Their recommendations are therefore heavily weighted towards regular review. For example, in 2004 they recommended routine screening for bacteriuria in pregnancy, in line with the NICE recommendations and a change from previous policy, and they have added screening for psychiatric illness in those with a previous history.

Table 4.1 NICE recommendations for antenatal screening

Condition	Screening	Comment
Haematological conditions		
Anaemia	Yes	At first appointment and at 28 weeks
Blood group + RhD status	Yes	Early in pregnancy, with follow-up as indicated
Fetal anomalies		
Structural anomalies	Yes	Ultrasound scan between 18 and 20 weeks
Down's syndrome	Yes	Using a test with current detection rate > 60% and false-positive rate < 5% (by April 2007 detection rate to rise to > 75% and false-positive rate to be < 3%)
Infections		
Asymptomatic bacteriuria	Yes	Early in pregnancy
Asymptomatic bacterial vaginosis	No	
Chlamydia trachomatis	No	May change with national screening programme
Cytomegalovirus	No	
Hepatitis B	Yes	Serological screening
Hepatitis C	No	Insufficient evidence
HIV	Yes	Early in pregnancy with clear referral paths for positive cases
Rubella	Yes	Early in pregnancy
Streptococcus group B	No	Evidence still uncertain
Syphilis	Yes	Early in pregnancy
Toxoplasmosis	No	Harm may outweigh benefit
Clinical conditions		
Gestational diabetes mellitus	No	
Pre-eclampsia		At first contact, risk of pre-eclampsia should be evaluated

The Antenatal Subgroup of the NSC has the following terms of reference:[5]

- to advise the NSC on the implementation, development, review, modification and, where necessary, the cessation of antenatal screening programmes
- to advise the NSC, the NHS Research and Development Programme (through its Standing Group on Health Technologies) and the Department of Health on the need for research reviews, for research in relation to antenatal screening, and for analytical work to help focus and make the best use of research
- to monitor and be advised of the progress, problems and research needs of ongoing antenatal screening programmes and, where appropriate, advise on standards and monitoring arrangements.

The NSC's position on antenatal screening is summarised in Table 4.2. As the national body charged with advising on screening policy, this must be regarded as the official Government position.

Table 4.2 The NSC's position on screening in the antenatal period

Disease	Current NSC policy	Comment
Anaemia	All pregnant women to be screened	To be reviewed in 2007
Bacteriuria in pregnancy	Should be offered routinely	To be reviewed in 2007
Bacterial vaginosis	Should not be offered routinely	To be reviewed in 2007
Blood group and RhD status and red cell alloantibodies	Testing should be offered for blood group and RhD status and screening for atypical red cell alloantibodies	To be reviewed in 2006
Chlamydia	Should not be offered routinely	To be reviewed in 2007
Cystic fibrosis	Not to be offered routinely at present despite the HTA recommendation	To be kept under review
Cytomegalovirus	ANSG review of the literature recommended against screening	Recommendation agreed by NSC – to be reviewed by March 2007
Diabetes	Should not be offered routinely	To be reviewed in 2006
Domestic violence	Should not be offered routinely	To be kept under review
Down's syndrome	Should be offered routinely. Model of best practice published	Ongoing implementation
Fetal anomalies	HTA systematic review of ultrasound screening found some advantage to a scan before 24 weeks	Ongoing review
Fetomaternal alloimmune thrombocytopenia	Not to be offered routinely	To be reviewed in 2006
Fragile X syndrome	On the basis of three HTA reports, not to be offered routinely	To be reviewed in 2007
Haemoglobinopathy, thalassaemia and sickle-cell disease	Should be offered routinely in high-prevalence areas by April 2004 (estimated fetal prevalence of >1.0 per 10 000). To start in low-prevalence areas from April 2004	To be kept under review
Haemolytic disease	Routine screening for rhesus incompatibility to be offered	To be reviewed by March 2006
Hepatitis B	Routine screening to be offered to identify infants who should be offered immunisation	To be reviewed in 2007
Hepatitis C	Not to be offered routinely	To be reviewed in 2006
Genital herpes	Not to be offered routinely	To be kept under review
HIV	To be offered to all pregnant women to reduce the rate of mother-to-child transmission	To be reviewed in 2007
HTLV1	Not to be offered routinely	To be reviewed in 2006
Neural-tube defect	Screening for spina bifida should be offered to all pregnant women	Ongoing review
Pre-eclampsia	Screening for risk factors for pre-eclampsia is part of routine antenatal care	To be reviewed following HTA report
Placenta praevia	Women with placenta praevia identified at 36 weeks should be offered a scan	To be reviewed in 2006
Psychiatric illness	Screening to be offered to women with a history of psychiatric illness	To be reviewed in 2007
Rubella immunity	Screening to continue	To be reviewed in 2007
Streptococcus B	Not to be offered routinely	Ongoing review
Syphilis	Universal screening to continue on the basis of a report from PHLS	To be reviewed in 2007
Tay–Sachs' disease	Screening supported by NSC in at-risk populations	To be reviewed in 2006
Thrombophilia	No evidence to support universal screening	To be reviewed in 2006
Toxoplasmosis	Not to be offered routinely	To be reviewed in 2007

RhD, rhesus factor; HTA, Health Technology Assessment; PHLS, Public Health Laboratory Service.

Table 4.3 Summary of antenatal screening in the UK for disorders that primarily affect the offspring

Disorder	Effective intervention?	Detection rate (%)	False-positive rate (%)	Is screening worthwhile?
Anencephaly	Yes	100	0	Yes
Cystic fibrosis	Yes	72	0.09	Yes
Down's syndrome	Yes	85	0.9	Yes
Duchenne muscular dystrophy	Yes	32	0.03	Probably
Fragile X syndrome	Yes	100	20	Possibly
Haemolytic disease				
anti-D	Yes	100	1.31	Yes
anti-K and anti-c	Yes	?	?	Probably
Haemophilia	Yes	55	< 0.01	Yes
Severe cardiac malformations	Yes	50	≤ 0.6	Yes
Spina bifida (open)	Yes	86	0.3	Yes
Tay–Sachs' disease	Yes	50	1	Yes
β-thalassaemia	Yes	89	7	Yes
X-linked retinitis pigmentosa	Yes	75	0.02	Possibly

Source: Simplified from Wald and Leck.[6] Reproduced by kind permission of the authors and Oxford University Press.

Table 4.4 Summary of antenatal screening in the UK for disorders of the offspring which are secondary to diseases in the mother

Disorder	Effective intervention?	Detection rate (%)	False-positive rate (%)	Is screening worthwhile?
Congenital syphilis	Yes	> 90	1.6	Probably
Rubella syndrome	Yes	> 90	1.6	Probably not
Sickle-cell disease	Yes	99	3	Yes
Vertically transmitted hepatitis B	Yes	≥ 98	0.14	Yes
Vertically transmitted HIV	Yes	99.9	0.13	Yes

Source: Simplified from Wald and Leck.[6] Reproduced by kind permission of the authors and Oxford University Press.

Wald and Leck's conclusions on the value of antenatal screening are summarised in Tables 4.3, 4.4 and 4.5.[6] However, in most of the conditions listed in Table 4.3 the only effective intervention is termination of pregnancy, an option which will not be acceptable for some. In all instances, it is crucial that the fullest information on what a positive screen would mean and a clear explanation of

Table 4.5 Summary of antenatal screening in the UK for specific disorders of the mother which may put the fetus at risk

Disorder	Is screening worthwhile?
Hyperglycaemia	Uncertain
Iron-deficiency anaemia	Yes
Thrombocytopenia	No

Source: Simplified from Wald and Leck.[6] Reproduced by kind permission of the authors and Oxford University Press.

the implications of the detection and false-positive rates are given to individuals and couples.

Wald and Leck stress that their recommendation on whether screening for a particular disorder is worthwhile is based on all the relevant factors, including the prevalence and severity of the condition, the success of screening, and the availability of an effective and acceptable intervention. The final assessment is a 'judgement over which there may be legitimate differences of opinion.'

These three authoritative sources[4–6] make clear the need for constant review and updating on antenatal screening and an overwhelming requirement to invoke the well-established screening criteria. There should also be a national consensus on antenatal screening so that tests and investigations are provided equitably across the country. Recommendations will inevitably change over time because of advances in knowledge and techniques, but also because of changes in the attitudes and norms of society.

Marteau and Dormandy[7] have drawn attention to the poor quality of much of the information provided to women undergoing antenatal testing. There is agreement that women and their partners need information on the condition for which testing is being offered, on the characteristics of the test itself, and on the implications of possible test results. From other studies they conclude that information provided about the condition tends to be brief and often negative, and they call for further research into this area: 'Thirty years after the routine introduction of prenatal diagnostic tests, we remain unaware how women are counselled, the information and support they receive, and how this affects the quality and type of decisions they make.'[7]

Routine screening

The antenatal period is usually taken to last from the beginning of pregnancy until the birth. It can also include the pre-conceptual period, particularly in diabetics and certain high-risk family and ethnic groups. In practical terms, however, it seems unlikely that most couples would seek screening before conception unless they were specifically advised to do so because of a known high level of risk.

Alderson and colleagues[8] have called for care in the use of terminology, in particular to avoid confusion between antenatal/prenatal and genetic screening. They contend that genetic screening – in its most precise sense of mass screening of asymptomatic groups for heritable genetic conditions confirmed by DNA analysis in pregnancy – does not yet occur in Europe, although it is often discussed as if it is already in common use. They conclude that the misleading use of the term 'genetic screening' opens the way for antenatal screening to become genetic without debate about whether societies, practitioners and prospective parents wish to take this step.

Fitzpatrick[9] also laments the influence of health scares on pregnant women. He cites a Department of Health pamphlet,[10] available without charge at antenatal clinics, which lists some of the hazards of pregnancy, including listeria (from cheese), toxoplasmosis (from cats), salmonella (from eggs) and chlamydia (from sheep). It gives detailed advice on how to avoid these infections, then comments that they are all 'very rare and it is unlikely that you or your baby will be affected.' If this is so, one has to wonder why it is felt necessary to highlight them in this way and subject the mainly healthy pregnant population to needless anxiety. Health scares, of which this is just one example, have acquired a virtually continuous presence in society and coexist with what Fitzpatrick describes as an 'unprecedented level of free-floating anxiety about health.'[9]

There currently seems to be agreement that antenatal screening for anaemia, bacteriuria, rhesus incompatibility, structural anomalies (e.g. spina bifida and cardiac abnormalities), Down's syndrome, hepatitis B, HIV, rubella immunity and syphilis should be offered to all women attending clinics in the UK. Serological screening early in pregnancy together with an ultrasound scan between 18 and 20 weeks would seem to be the method of choice in most of these conditions, with subsequent diagnostic testing as appropriate. It cannot be emphasised too often that such screening should only be offered if adequate counselling and follow-up services are available.

Ultrasound scanning

Since its introduction in the 1980s, fetal ultrasound scanning has become routine practice in many western countries. A survey in 1996 in the UK[11] reported that 82% of maternity units now offer such a scan, usually at about 18 weeks of pregnancy. The original goal of scanning was to reduce obstetric risk by correcting gestational age, locating the placenta and diagnosing multiple pregnancies. As imaging technology has developed there has been an increasing emphasis on fetal diagnosis of structural anomalies such as anencephaly and spina bifida. Disclosure of more subtle anomalies such as cleft lip is also now possible.

However, as Getz and Kirkengen point out,[12] the net medical benefits of ultrasound screening, measured in terms of maternal and fetal mortality and morbidity, are still open to debate. One clinician conducting fetal ultrasound scanning on a routine basis described the uncertainty of her work as like 'walking blindfold in tiger country.'[13]

There is a need to pay close attention to the crucial distinction between technology development and technology implementation in relation to antenatal screening. One of the concerns is the current trend towards supplementing or replacing second-trimester ultrasound with ultrasound screening between gestational weeks 11 and 14, and the use of so-called anatomical soft markers.

Soft markers are defined as 'structural changes detected at ultrasound scan which may be transient and in themselves have little or no pathological significance, but are thought to be more commonly found in fetuses with congenital abnormalities, particularly karyotypic abnormalities.'[14]

Getz and Kirkengen conclude that their analysis of the published biomedical literature makes it clear that the 'practice of routine fetal screening by obstetrical ultrasound applying the latest in diagnostic equipment has caused harm to an unknown number of expectant parents and unborn children during the last decade.'[12] Many examiners have counselled pregnant women about an increased risk of fetal chromosomal aberrations on the basis of subtle findings in the ultrasonographic image which have not subsequently been substantiated.

As these researchers state, 'Profound and private moral dilemmas arise as a direct consequence of premature application of an advancing medical technology in a routine clinical setting.'[12]

On the other hand, the pleasure of women in seeing their baby for the first time and then being able to follow its development by ultrasound should not be discounted. It is common for expectant mothers to show off a print of an ultrasound image.

On the basis of a review of published studies, the Canadian Preventive Services Task Force found fair evidence for including a single ultrasound examination in the second trimester in women without clinical indications.[15] There was no statistically significant effect of screening on live births or Apgar scores, but screening appeared to result in increased birth weight, earlier detection of twins, decreased rates of induction and increased rates of abortion for fetal abnormalities. With regard to serial ultrasound in the second and third trimesters in normal pregnancies, there was no evidence of improved perinatal mortality or morbidity. The Task Force emphasised the need for further research into the benefits and disadvantages of ultrasound examination, including the psychological effects of screening on the parents.

The US Preventive Services Task Force does not recommend routine ultrasound examination in the third trimester, concluding that it shows no benefit for either the pregnant woman or her fetus.[16] They stress that this applies to routine ultrasonography, not to diagnostic ultrasonography for specific clinical indications.

Table 4.6 Specified abnormality scanning: categories of benefit

Benefit from screening by ultrasound	Possible or no benefit from screening by ultrasound
Abnormalities associated with serious disability for which termination of pregnancy is justifiable	Abnormalities for which there is a possible benefit in antenatal identification but no clear evidence as to whether this is so
Fetal abnormalities for which termination of pregnancy avoids continuing with an unproductive pregnancy	Abnormalities for which there is no benefit in antenatal identification
Abnormalities for which *in-utero* treatment reduces morbidity	
Abnormalities for which immediate postnatal treatment reduces morbidity	

In their approach to ultrasound screening, Wald and colleagues[17] advocate what they describe as *specified abnormality scanning*. This entails scanning only for abnormalities for which antenatal screening confers benefit that outweighs harm and cost. They identify four categories of congenital abnormalities in which there is such benefit, and two where there is not. These categories are summarised in Table 4.6.

In order to obtain genuine consent, women should be given full information on the various disorders involved, explaining for each the implications of a positive screening test, the further tests and interventions that might be offered and the possible consequences of not intervening. Women who would not consider termination of pregnancy for conditions on the list could choose not to be informed of the findings for these conditions or decline to have an ultrasound scan for fetal abnormalities. Screening for abnormalities for which no intervention can be offered is unjustified:

> Doing so simply to prepare parents before the birth is not helpful. If no intervention is to be offered, the psychological cost of an uncertain prognosis, or in the case of minor abnormalities an excessive pre-occupation with the condition, can easily outweigh any benefits of being prepared, and this is not a sound basis for a screening investigation.[17]

Wald and colleagues[17] also stress that the application of specified abnormality scanning will require further discussion, education and examination of data to determine which disorders should be specified.

It seems, therefore, that the jury on ultrasound scanning is still out and that, although high-quality scanning can identify abnormalities in certain pregnancies, it can also cause harm by prompting anxiety and unnecessary medical intervention. Many of the so-called abnormalities identified by ultrasound screening are not significant and do not meet screening criteria. For most women a high-quality ultrasound scan between 18 and 20 weeks as recommended by NICE, to confirm gestational age and identify multiple births and key specified anomalies, would seem sensible.

Down's syndrome

Down's syndrome is the commonest chromosomal abnormality associated with significant risk of long-term morbidity. The primary objective of antenatal screening for this condition is to allow parents the choice of whether to continue with an affected pregnancy or have it terminated. It is therefore aimed at secondary rather than primary prevention. Other benefits include reassurance that the baby is normal or the opportunity to adjust to Down's syndrome before the birth. Disadvantages include the risk of fetal loss after invasive diagnostic tests and the problems arising from false-positive and false-negative results.

In April 2001, the UK Government announced that it had accepted the National Screening Committee's recommendation that all pregnant women, irrespective of age, should be offered second-trimester serum screening for Down's syndrome: 'The test used should comprise at least a double test, but it would be desirable for laboratories to move to triple or quadruple tests when possible.' Its aim is to increase the antenatal detection rate for Down's syndrome and to reduce the amniocentesis rate with its associated hazards. A network of regional co-ordinators is currently being set up across the country to ensure proper management of local programmes, but with no resources for quality control. Since March 2004, the performance standard has been a detection rate of at least 60%, with a false-positive rate of 3% or less.

Although this ends the previous piecemeal approach in which policies on screening varied from region to region in the UK,[18] there are those who contend that this strategy has underlying social, ethical and legal hazards that have not been widely debated.[19]

As Alderson has stated:

> Choice may load women with responsibility, guilt and blame. To refuse [the test] may appear to be casual, even callous; to accept the birth of an impaired child, expected or not, can look like a selfish extravagance and may become a lonely burden.[20]

Wellesley and colleagues[21] conducted a six-year retrospective study in the maternity units of eight district general hospitals to compare the effectiveness of different screening policies for the antenatal detection of Down's syndrome. Serum and nuchal translucency screening have been widely introduced without controlled trials of their effectiveness, and these workers found no evidence that such screening improves the antenatal detection rates or reduces the subsequent need for invasive procedures. They also drew attention to the uncertainty about the best way to screen for Down's syndrome because of the lack of clear evidence, with the eight district general hospitals within one health region using seven different policies.

Wald and colleagues[22] contend that this study ignored evidence from previous work showing the substantial advantage of serum screening over screening based on maternal age alone. They also rejected the call for controlled trials. Christiansen and colleagues[23] claim that the study's conclusion contradicts international experience, and that it cannot be reached on the basis of the data reported.

In response to these criticisms, Howe and Wellesley stood by their recommendation that screening programmes should be tested in controlled trials before implementation, and emphasised that the purpose of their study was to audit screening in day-to-day practice, where 'theory is disrupted by reality. In this reality women choose not to behave as expected, hence screening programmes do not perform as predicted by theoretical models.'[24]

Smith and colleagues[25] have previously drawn attention to the gap between policy and practice in obtaining informed consent for serum screening for Down's syndrome. They stressed that the decision as to whether or not to undergo screening must be made by the pregnant woman on the basis of sound information. They also suggested that more effective staff training for healthcare professionals on how to promote truly informed decision making, including information on possible adverse outcomes, was needed. Whether that training has been provided in the 10 years since the publication of their paper is not clear.

Second-trimester maternal serum screening can effectively detect around 60% of Down's syndrome fetuses. Although it is now possible to detect the anomaly earlier, using first-trimester serum and ultrasound markers, this would expose more parents to the need to make difficult decisions about the termination of a pregnancy that might otherwise have miscarried spontaneously. Chitty[26] therefore concluded that second-trimester serum screening should be used until the results of further evaluation of earlier diagnosis become available.

Wald and colleagues[27] assessed the performance of antenatal serum screening for Down's syndrome with the quadruple test in 46 193 pregnancies from 14 hospitals over a period of five years.* The test had a detection rate of 81% and a false-positive rate of 7%. Using maternal age alone, the detection rate would have been much lower, at 51%, and the false-positive rate would have been twice as high (14%). On the basis of these results, they concluded that the quadruple test should be regarded as the screening test of choice in the second trimester.

Across the Atlantic, official opinion of screening for Down's syndrome is broadly in line with government policy in the UK.

Dick, in his review for the Canadian Preventive Services Task Force,[28] concluded that there is fair evidence for including prenatal diagnosis with amniocentesis or chorionic villus sampling for women aged over 35 years, those with a previous Down's syndrome birth and those with a known family history. He also suggests that there is a benefit in offering second-trimester triple-marker serum screening to pregnant women under 35 years of age, with appropriate information to enable informed choice.

The second edition of the US Guide to Clinical Preventive Services, *Screening for Down Syndrome*,[29] recommends that amniocentesis and chorionic villus sampling should be offered to high-risk pregnant women. Screening by serum multiple markers is recommended for all low-risk pregnant women and as an alternative first option to amniocentesis and chorionic villus sampling for high-risk women. The authors stress that this testing should only be offered to women who are seen for prenatal care in locations that have adequate counselling and follow-up services.

Roizen and Patterson,[30] in an overview of the screening and management of Down's syndrome, call for research efforts to further improve the sensitivity and specificity of screening for the condition to reduce the number of women who require an invasive diagnostic test, or ideally eliminate them altogether.

Wald[31] reiterates that the ability of the mother to choose is an essential element of screening. In general terms, about 70% of women accept the offer of antenatal screening for Down's syndrome, and about 70% of those with a positive screening result decide to undergo a diagnostic amniocentesis or chorionic villus sampling. Over 90% of those with a positive diagnostic result then opt for a termination of pregnancy. He states that it is reasonable to estimate that about 50% of affected pregnancies will be identified and result in a therapeutic abortion.

Wald and Canick[32] have also drawn attention to the difficulty that arises when the method of screening for one disorder additionally identifies another that would not justify screening in its own right. They cite the identification of trisomy 18 as part of antenatal screening for Down's syndrome as an example of this, and they caution that the 'case for seeking other disorders within screening programmes needs to be evaluated as rigorously as the primary programme.'[32]

It seems clear that although the offer of serum screening for Down's syndrome

---

* The quadruple test calculates the risk of a Down's syndrome term pregnancy from maternal age at term and the concentration of four markers in maternal serum.

made to all pregnant women is now accepted health policy in the UK as well as widely elsewhere, attention must be paid to the issue of truly informed choice. Although healthcare professionals in specialised research centres may be offering full and rounded information on the benefits and possible harms of screening, we need to ensure that this level of expertise is being transferred into antenatal practice in the routine clinical setting. For example, are all women given full information on exactly what conditions the serum sample they provide at the antenatal clinic will be looking for or, as seems more likely, will the sample be taken under the general remit of 'seeing that everything is all right?' There also remain major postcode differences in what is available, and in equality of access.

In the information that is given to mothers it is important to emphasise that the prognosis of Down's syndrome is now different from that of 20 years ago. Methods of treatment for associated defects, such as congenital heart disease, have improved. Many individuals with the syndrome are educable and can pursue a productive life, although this of course depends on the severity of the condition, which cannot be predicted.

Conclusion

Our recommendations on screening in the antenatal period are summarised in Table 4.7.

Two issues, both mentioned earlier in the chapter, cannot be overemphasised in this context. First, we must take care not to medicalise this normal stage of life where most pregnancies have a successful outcome. Our current media-fuelled preoccupation with health must not be allowed to taint pregnancy and birth.

Secondly, there must be full, balanced and understandable information available for pregnant women, and properly trained healthcare professionals with time to provide and/or explain it. This is important for all pregnant women, but particularly for the minority who are unfortunate enough to experience difficulty and defect.

Neonatal screening

Screening procedures in the period immediately after birth and in the first months of life can be divided into those that are part of routine screening for all newborn babies either by clinical examination or biochemical tests, and those conditions such as hearing loss that will require separate testing.

Routine bloodspot screening is recommended for phenylketonuria, congenital hypothyroidism (and galactosaemia in Scotland) and cystic fibrosis, with screening for thalassaemia and sickle-cell disease currently being introduced for all newborn babies. The UK Newborn Screening Programme Centre was established in 2002 with a remit to monitor and improve the quality of newborn bloodspot screening procedures and their outcomes for parents and their babies.

The routine physical examination will cover congenital heart disease, congenital malformations, congenital cataract and cryptorchidism. The Child Health Subgroup of the NSC is currently looking at standards and variability of quality in this area, and a training programme on newborn physical examination is under

Table 4.7 Our recommendations for screening in the antenatal period

Routine		
Asymptomatic bacteriuria		
Risk factors for pre-eclampsia		
Anaemia		
Blood group and RhD status		
Hepatitis B	Blood test	Early in pregnancy with effective follow-up for any abnormalities identified
HIV		
Rubella immunity		
Syphilis		
Fetal anomalies		
Anencephaly	Ultrasound and blood test if indicated	Between 18 and 20 weeks with effective follow-up
Spina bifida		
Chromosome abnormalities	Quadruple serum tests and ultrasound	Second trimester with effective follow-up
Down's syndrome		
High risk only		
Thalassaemia/sickle-cell disease		
Tay–Sachs' disease		
Under research review		
Duchenne muscular dystrophy		
Chlamydia		
Gestational diabetes		
Fragile X syndrome		
Hepatitis C		
Genital herpes		
HTLV1		
Streptococcus B		

development to try to ensure uniformity.[33] For hearing, universal newborn screening has now been rolled out over most of the UK.

The NSC's recommendations for screening in the neonatal period are shown in Tables 4.8 and 4.9.

Bloodspot screening

Two prime candidates for neonatal screening are phenylketonuria and congenital hypothyroidism. Screening for cystic fibrosis remains more contentious, but a national programme is currently being introduced in the UK.

Table 4.8 The NSC's position on neonatal bloodspot screening

Condition	Current NSC policy	Comment
Biotinidase deficiency	Not to be offered routinely	To be kept under review
Congenital adrenal hyperplasia	Not to be offered routinely	To be kept under review
Congenital hypothyroidism Phenylketonuria	Routine	Ongoing
Cystic fibrosis	Universal screening to be phased in	Update ongoing
Duchenne muscular dystrophy	Not to be offered routinely	To be kept under review
Sickle-cell disease	Screening being introduced for all newborns	Update ongoing
Medium-chain acyl CoA dehydrogenase deficiency (MCADD)	Not to be offered at present – evaluative study commissioned	To be kept under review

Table 4.9 The NSC's position on other neonatal screening

Condition	Current NSC policy	Comment
Biliary atresia	Not to be offered routinely	To be kept under review
Congenital heart disease	Part of the routine physical examination of newborn babies	Update in progress
Congenital cataract	Part of the routine physical examination of newborn babies	Update ongoing
Congenital malformations, including congenital dislocation of the hip	Part of the routine physical examination of newborn babies	Update ongoing
Cryptorchidism	Part of the routine physical examination of newborn babies	Update ongoing
Hearing	Universal newborn screening has been rolled out over most of the UK	Ongoing
Neonatal alloimmune thrombocytopenia	Not to be offered routinely	
Neuroblastoma	Not to be offered at present	To be kept under review

Phenylketonuria and congenital hypothyroidism

Blood-based screening of newborn babies for phenylketonuria was recommended as a national programme by the Department of Health in 1969, and this was the beginning of modern neonatal screening. It had been introduced in Scotland four years earlier, and covered the whole of the country by 1968.

As Cunningham states,[34] phenylketonuria has been described as the 'epitome of metabolic disease screening.' If left untreated, the condition (which has an expected incidence of 10–25 per 100 000 live births*) has serious consequences, the most important of which is progressive mental retardation, often with associated neurological damage. The mechanics of the condition are well understood,[35] and there is a suitable diagnostic test which is available, safe and acceptable. Phenylketonuria can be very successfully treated, essentially by diet.

Congenital hypothyroidism is another condition that has been part of the routine screening programme for all newborn babies since 1981.[36] Although it is relatively uncommon (expected incidence 25 per 100 000 births), the consequences for an untreated baby are serious. Effective treatment is available and should be started within four weeks of birth.

The UK screening programmes for phenylketonuria and congenital hypothyroidism are long established, have largely achieved their expected objectives and are cost-effective.[37] Current concerns include 'the difficulties of maintaining adequate coverage, perceived organisational weakness and a lack of overview.'

Cystic fibrosis (CF)

The prevalence of cystic fibrosis in the UK is about 1 per 2500 live births, but it is especially common in Northern Ireland (1 in 1850 live births). It is an unpleasant condition that affects mainly the pancreas and lungs and causes chest infections and poor digestion. Treatment is primarily symptomatic, but can help to maintain good nutrition and minimise chest infections with improved quality of life and life expectancy.

As Dezateux has pointed out,[38] there is still ambiguity about whether screening for this disorder should be performed in the antenatal or neonatal period.

In 1998, Wald and Morris[39] reported on the results of an American randomised controlled trial of neonatal screening which involved two-thirds of a million newborn infants and their follow-up.[40] Although the study showed that screening and subsequent treatment improved the growth and development of children with cystic fibrosis, Wald and Morris commented that this may not be justified because of some problems with the analysis of the data. They suggested that current evidence is not encouraging and does not warrant a change in policy from that suggested by the 1997 NIH Consensus Statement that 'offering cystic fibrosis genetic testing to newborn infants is not recommended.'

In 1999, Murray and colleagues recommended the introduction of antenatal screening in the UK, but were unable to make a similar recommendation for neonatal screening.[41] They recommended that more research should be under-

---

* The UK average is 11.0, with wide geographical variation, and there is a particularly high incidence in Northern Ireland.

taken on neonatal screening and stressed the importance of good information in order to obtain truly informed consent from parents.

Despite the doubts, in 2001 the UK Public Health Minister announced the introduction of neonatal screening for cystic fibrosis in England and Wales, with a similar announcement for Scotland. An Implementation Group was set up to provide advice on screening protocol. Screening started throughout Scotland in February 2003, is also in place in Wales and Northern Ireland, and is now being implemented in England.

An update on the 1991 Cochrane Review of newborn screening for cystic fibrosis was published early in 2004.[42] On the basis of the data available, the reviewers concluded that nutritional benefits are apparent and that screening does provide a potential opportunity for better pulmonary outcomes. Additional analysis is ongoing.

Stewart and Oliver[43] stress that the need for better provision of information to parents before seeking informed consent for screening and more skilled communication of test results and genetic counselling are paramount in bloodspot screening in general, and for cystic fibrosis in particular. The Scottish Newborn Screening Laboratory has a well-established programme and screens approximately 52 000 newborn babies a year for phenylketonuria, congenital hypothyroidism and cystic fibrosis, with the aim of diagnosing these conditions as early as possible 'to allow affected infants to be placed upon the appropriate corrective treatment.' They produce an information pamphlet entitled *Parents' Guide to Newborn Screening for Phenylketonuria, Congenital Hypothyroidism and Cystic Fibrosis*, which gives clear details of the conditions, tests and treatments, as well as sources of additional information.[44]

There are those who remain sceptical. TJ David, a paediatrician who treats children with cystic fibrosis, suggests that the case made for neonatal screening for the condition was more political than scientific.[45] There is a lack of universal agreement about the best screening protocol, although the two-tier immunoreactive trypsin/DNA analysis proposed in the UK programme should be satisfactory.

The most consistently observed benefits of early diagnosis thus far have been nutritional, but the efficacy of screening in preventing lung damage is more difficult to demonstrate. Concerns about pre-symptomatic diagnosis by screening include possible harm caused by aggressive treatment with antibiotics and chest physiotherapy, and early cross-infection in clinics or wards from individuals with *Pseudomonas* lung infection.

Psychosocial harm caused by the way in which a positive screening result is handled is a further potential problem. There is a need in this context for a wide range of professional staff to provide the care and information required, yet many cystic fibrosis centres are chronically understaffed. There is also concern about possible adverse effects on infants identified as carriers of a CF gene mutation.

David concludes that a theoretical benefit from early diagnosis should be the enrolment of newly diagnosed patients into multi-centre randomised controlled trials of existing new treatment: 'In practice, the variation in treatment strategies in CF is huge – a legacy of the serious dearth of controlled trials of treatments – making large controlled trials hard to perform.'[45]

Farrell and Farrell[46] also acknowledge the potential for harm as well as benefit from screening for cystic fibrosis. They stress that screening identifies the opportunity to achieve good results but does not automatically lead to more good than harm. The potential benefits for cystic fibrosis screening using IRT/ DNA are compelling, but the key is excellent implementation with optimal follow-up care for all.

Given that neonatal screening for cystic fibrosis is now a reality in the UK, scientific evaluation of actual delivery must be a priority.

Routine clinical examination

As mentioned above, a routine clinical examination is carried out on all newborn babies in the UK and this should, in theory, identify congenital and other abnormalities that can then be more fully investigated. The Child Health Subgroup of the NSC, in an effort to reduce variability in quality across the country, is developing a training programme on newborn physical examination, which is often carried out by relatively junior doctors.

Congenital dislocation of the hip/developmental dysplasia of the hip

Possible congenital malformations include congenital dislocation of the hip (CDH). Universal clinical screening for CDH, through detection of neonatal hip instability, was introduced in the UK in 1969.[47] It is thus long established, but is still a cause of debate and concern.[48,49]

The recent change in nomenclature from CDH to developmental dysplasia of the hip (DDH) illustrates the complexity of the condition and the range of anatomical and clinical abnormalities covered.

Screening guidelines for CDH rather than DDH were updated in 1986.[50] The reasoning then was that early detection would allow prompt management and reduce the need for later surgery. The Ortolani manoeuvre and the Barlow tests are used to examine every newborn baby in the UK. The recommendation was to screen three times during the first 6 weeks of life (within 24 hours of birth, on discharge from hospital and at the age of 6 weeks). Clinical examination for classic signs of dislocation and abnormal gait was advised until walking age. A national survey in 1994 showed that this remained current practice at that time.[51]

The specificity of these tests is high but their sensitivity can be low, depending upon who performs them. Since treatment requires confirmation by ultrasound examination, the problem is missing cases rather than over-treatment.

Ultrasound examination can be offered to those identified by initial screening, but again there can be difficulties with false-positive results and over-treatment in those whose hip instability may resolve spontaneously.

Holen and colleagues reported a prospective randomised trial of 15 500 newborn babies to compare population and selective screening programmes.[52] With a follow-up period of between 6 and 11 years, they found no additional benefit from universal screening.

In Germany, a national hip ultrasound screening programme, undertaken during the first 6 weeks of life, was introduced in 1996 and continued for 5 years.[53] The results indicated that although the programme was successful in reducing the rate of operations, improvements were needed in the timing of the procedure and in training doctors in the assessment of ultrasound images. It was concluded that better-quality data for conservative treatment rates for DDH are needed in order to monitor and possibly reduce over-treatment.

In the UK, a population-based screening programme has been running in Coventry for 13 years. In total, 98% of babies are screened at birth; 6% have abnormalities and attend for further scans and/or treatment as required. No late diagnosis has been identified in a screened baby.[54] Although good practice in a single locality is not representative of the national picture, it would be foolish to ignore these results in any reassessment of the current screening programme.

The MRC Working Group on Congenital Dislocation of the Hip looked at the picture again and reported in 1998.[55] They stressed the importance of continued vigilant observation of hips and gait throughout infancy and early childhood, with the role of parents as well as healthcare professionals being crucial. They drew attention to the difficulties created by the introduction of the national programme before recognised criteria for screening were met, and they pointed to substantial variation nationally both in screening and management practices and in outcome.

They concluded that a formal comparison is needed of the effectiveness of existing and alternative screening policies, including universal primary ultrasound examination of the newborn hip.

In 2002, the UK Collaborative Hip Trial Group reported on a study to assess clinical effectiveness and the net cost of ultrasound examination compared with clinical assessment alone, to provide guidance for the management of infants with clinical hip instability.[56] They found that the use of ultrasound examination allowed abduction splinting rates to be reduced and was not associated with an increase in abnormal hip development, higher rates of surgical treatment by 2 years of age or significantly higher health service costs.

In her review of neonatal hip screening, Eastwood highlights the problem that ultrasound examination of the infant hip identifies so-called abnormalities whose significance is unknown: 'Are these dysplastic cases simply immature hips that will mature unaided? Is this the ultrasound equivalent of the clinical hip instability which is present at birth but gone by 2 weeks?'[57] She concludes that the effectiveness of screening for CDH/DDH still needs to be established: 'We must define what we are screening for, who is going to do it and who is going to provide treatment . . . .Until we have defined and established a successful programme, cost-effectiveness cannot be considered.'[57]

Perhaps we should be looking to the Coventry programme[54] as a national model.

Hearing impairment

Neonatal hearing screening has been in place in the UK since the early 1960s using the Health Visitor Distraction Test. The main problem with this is that the test does not have high sensitivity or specificity, so many infants have either been subjected to unnecessary follow-up or have not had their impairment identified. It also has the disadvantage that, because it is a test of behaviour and requires the infant to show a reaction to sound, it cannot be used in children under 6 months of age.

There is growing evidence for the benefits of early identification of a hearing impairment, both in terms of developing language and social skills and in providing support for parents. And the technology now exists to screen a baby's hearing within a few hours of birth.[58]

In 1999, the Children's Subgroup of the NSC recommended the introduction of universal neonatal hearing screening, and a national Newborn Hearing Screening Programme (NHSP) has now been established.[59]

This uses two types of test. The most common type is the oto-acoustic emission test (OAE), which takes only a few minutes while the baby is asleep. It is not always possible to obtain a clear response from this in very young babies, and in these cases the method of choice is the automated auditory brainstem response (AABR). Both methods are very safe and effective ways to check for signs of possible hearing impairment.

The programme began in England with 20 pilot sites, using the OAE as the primary screening test, and has now been rolled out over most of the UK. Complete coverage should be achieved by 2005. In Scotland two pathfinder sites were set up in Lothian and Tayside NHS Boards to start the programme and establish quality standards.

Conclusion

Our recommendations for screening in the neonatal period are summarised in Table 4.10.

The training programme that is being developed for those who undertake the routine clinical examination of newborn babies should help to ensure that

Table 4.10 Our recommendations for screening in the neonatal period

Condition	Comment
Routine	
Bloodspot for	
Phenylketonuria	Must be properly evaluated
Congenital hypothyroidism	In process of introduction for all newborns
Cystic fibrosis	
Sickle-cell disease	
Physical examination	Training programme in physical
Congenital heart disease	examination being developed
Congenital cataract	
Cryptorchidism	
Congenital dislocation of the hip/	Use of ultrasound as primary screening test
developmental dysplasia of the hip	to be evaluated
Other congenital malformations	
Other tests	
Hearing impairment	Implementation ongoing
Under research review	
Biotinidase deficiency	
Congenital adrenal hyperplasia	
Duchenne muscular dystrophy	

variations in quality are minimised. Relatively inexperienced doctors are often expected to perform this task, and it is vital that it is carried out to the highest standards. Topics covered should include skills for communication with parents. Of course it is desirable to identify abnormalities as soon as possible when they can be treated or alleviated, but the harm-to-benefit ratio is particularly important at this early stage. The value of accurate and understandable information that is communicated well cannot be overstated.

The contribution that antenatal and neonatal screening can make to the prevention of disability has been estimated by Wald and Leck.[6] They identified two groups of disorders – first, severe congenital abnormalities which cannot be treated but in which termination of pregnancy can be offered, and secondly, conditions in which early diagnosis can allow effective treatment (*see* Table 4.11).

Table 4.11 Estimate of severe childhood disability preventable by screening in the UK

Disorder	Preventable cases of handicap (per 10 000 births)
Conditions in which termination of pregnancy is an option	
Cystic fibrosis	2.5
Down's syndrome	14
Duchenne muscular dystrophy	0.45
Fragile X syndrome	1.2
Haemophilia	0.3
Rubella syndrome	0.03
Spina bifida (open)	3
Tay–Sachs' disease	0.02
β-thalassaemia	5
Subtotal	26
Conditions in which children can be enabled to survive without handicap	
Congenital dislocation of the hip	7
Congenital hypothyroidism	3
Congenital syphilis	0.15
Galactosaemia due to absence of transferase	0.15
Haemolytic disease	2
Phenylketonuria	1
Sickle-cell disease	3
Vertically transmitted HIV infection	0.6
Subtotal	17
Total	43 (approximately 17% of severe childhood disability that would occur without screening)

Source: Reproduced by kind permission of the authors and Oxford University Press.[6]

In conclusion, there are five points to be remembered about screening at this early stage of life.

First, although screening can make a valuable contribution to preventive medicine, it can only prevent a minority of deaths and disabilities. This highlights the importance of traditional postnatal medical services to identify and treat congenital, orthopaedic and cardiac abnormalities.

Secondly, most of the recent benefits in antenatal and neonatal screening have arisen from the better use of existing knowledge and the improved application of techniques (e.g. ultrasound) that have been available for over 20 years.

Thirdly, there is a continuing need to avoid generating unreasonable expectations with regard to the value of molecular biology and genome mapping in antenatal screening. Now that gene-specific probes are being identified for an increasing number of conditions, problems concerning their relevance as general population screening tests are coming into sharper focus. As was discussed in Chapter 2, genetic biochemistry may identify very rare conditions for which there is no treatment, and there is also the possibility of false-positive results leading to unjustified termination of pregnancy. This type of screening must be rigorously evaluated to proven criteria, and should not be proposed solely because a test is available.

Fourthly, as in every screening programme, good information effectively imparted is crucial in allowing parents to make a truly informed choice.

Finally, despite initiatives such as the establishment of the NSC and the National Newborn Screening Programme Centre, which have undoubtedly resulted in substantial progress, much remains to be done to improve the organisation and equity of antenatal and neonatal screening services across the country.

References

1 Doll R (2000) Foreword. In: N Wald and I Leck (eds) *Antenatal and Neonatal Screening* (2e). Oxford University Press, Oxford.

2 House of Commons Social Services Committee (1980) *Report on Perinatal and Neonatal Mortality*. HMSO, London.

3 Jewell D (1992) Antenatal and postnatal care. In: CR Hart and P Burke (eds) *Screening and Surveillance in General Practice*. Churchill Livingstone, Edinburgh.

4 National Institute for Clinical Excellence (NICE) (2003) *Antenatal Care. Routine care for the healthy pregnant woman*. Clinical Guideline 6. NICE, London.

5 UK National Screening Committee's Antenatal Subgroup; www.nsc.nhs.uk/

6 Wald N and Leck I (2000) Conclusions. In: N Wald and I Leck (eds) *Antenatal and Neonatal Screening* (2e). Oxford University Press, Oxford.

7 Marteau TM and Dormandy E (2001) Facilitating informed choice in prenatal testing: how well are we doing? *Am J Med Genet.* **106**: 185–90.

8 Alderson P, Arja AR, Dragonas T *et al.* (2001) Prenatal screening and genetics. *Eur J Public Health.* **11**: 231–3.

9 Fitzpatrick M (2001) *The Tyranny of Health*. Routledge, London.

10 Department of Health (1991) *While You Are Pregnant*. HMSO, London.

11 Royal College of Obstetricians and Gynaecologists/Royal College of Radiologists (RCOG/RCR) (1996) *Survey on the Use of Obstetric Ultrasound in the UK. Report of the RCOG Working Party on Ultrasound Screening for Fetal Abnormalities*. Consultation Document. RCOG/RCR, London.

12 Getz L and Kirkengen AL (2003) Ultrasound screening in pregnancy: advancing technology, soft markers for fetal chromosomal aberrations and unacknowledged ethical dilemmas. *Soc Sci Med.* **56**: 2045–57.

13 Furness ME (1987) Reporting obstetric ultrasound. *Lancet.* **1**: 675–6.

14 Bricker L, Garcia J, Henderson J *et al.* (2000) Ultrasound screening in pregnancy: a systematic review of the clinical effectiveness, cost-effectiveness and women's views. *Health Technol Assess.* **4**(16).

15 Anderson G (1994) Routine prenatal ultrasound screening. In: *Canadian Guide to Clinical Preventive Health Care*. Canada Communication Group, Ottawa.

16 US Preventive Services Task Force (1996) *Screening Ultrasonography in Pregnancy. Guide to clinical preventive services* (2e); http://cpmcnet.columbia.edu/texts/gcps/

17 Wald N, Kennard A, Donnenfeld A and Leck I (2000) Ultrasound scanning for congenital abnormalities. In: N Wald and I Leck (eds) *Antenatal and Neonatal Screening* (2e). Oxford University Press, Oxford.

18 MacIntosh M, Ellis A, Cuckle H and Seth J (1998) Variation in biochemical screening for Down's syndrome in the United Kingdom. *Br J Obstet Gynaecol.* **105**: 465–7.

19 Robins JB (2002) *Prenatal screening for Down's syndrome: right or wrong?* MPhil Thesis, University of Glasgow, Glasgow.

20 Alderson P (2001) Prenatal screening ethics and Down's syndrome. A literature review. *Nurs Ethics.* **8**: 360–74.

21 Wellesley D, Boyle T, Barber J and Howe DT (2002) Retrospective audit of different antenatal screening policies for Down's syndrome in eight district general hospitals in one health region. *BMJ.* **325**: 15.

22 Wald NJ, Huttly W and Hackshaw AK (2002) Antenatal screening policies for Down's syndrome (letter). *BMJ.* **325**: 1034.

23 Christiansen M, Larsen SO and Norgaard-Pedersen B (2002) Serum screening for Down's syndrome is better than age screening (letter). *BMJ.* **325**: 1034.

24 Howe D and Wellesley D (2002) Authors' reply (letter). *BMJ.* **325**: 1034.

25 Smith DK, Shaw RW and Marteau TM (1994) Informed consent to undergo serum screening for Down's syndrome: the gap between policy and practice. *BMJ.* **309**: 776.

26 Chitty L (1998) Screening for chromosome abnormalities. *Br Med Bull.* **54**: 839–56.

27 Wald NJ, Huttly W and Hackshaw AK (2003) Antenatal screening for Down's syndrome with the quadruple test. *Lancet.* **361**: 835–6.

28 Dick P (1994) Prenatal screening and diagnosis for Down syndrome prevention. In: *Canadian Guide to Clinical Preventive Health Care*. Canada Communication Group, Ottawa.

29 US Preventive Services Task Force (1996) *Screening for Down Syndrome. Guide to clinical preventive services* (2e); http://cpmcnet.columbia.edu/texts/gcps/

30 Roizen NJ and Patterson D (2003) Down's syndrome. *Lancet.* **361**: 1281–9.

31 Wald N (2000) Down's syndrome. In: N Wald and I Leck (eds) *Antenatal and Neonatal Screening* (2e). Oxford University Press, Oxford.

32 Wald NJ and Canick JA (2002) Seeking other disorders within antenatal serum screening programmes for Down's syndrome. *J Med Screen.* **9**: 145–6.

33 Child Health Screening Subgroup of the UK National Screening Committee; www.nsc.nhs.uk/

34 Cunningham GC (2000) Phenylketonuria and other inherited metabolic defects. In: N Wald and I Leck (eds) *Antenatal and Neonatal Screening* (2e). Oxford University Press, Oxford.

35 Scriver CR and Clow CL (1980) Phenylketonuria. Epitome of biochemical genetics. *NEJM.* **303**: 1336–400.

36 Pollitt R *et al.* (1997) Neonatal screening for inborn errors of metabolism: a review. *Health Technol Assess.* **1**(7).

37 Seymour CA *et al.* (1997) Neonatal screening for inborn errors of metabolism: a systematic review. *Health Technol Assess.* **1**(11).

38 Dezateux C (2001) Screening newborn infants for cystic fibrosis (editorial). *J Med Screen.* **8**: 57–60.

39 Wald N and Morris JK (1998) Neonatal screening for cystic fibrosis (editorial). *BMJ.* **316**: 404–5.

40 Farrell PM, Kosorok MR, Rock MJ *et al.* (2001) Early diagnosis of cystic fibrosis through neonatal screening prevents severe malnutrition and improves long-term growth. Wisconsin Cystic Fibrosis Neonatal Screening Study Group. *Pediatrics.* **107**: 1–13.

41 Murray J, Cuckle H, Taylor G, Littlewood J and Hewison J (1999) Screening for cystic fibrosis. *Health Technol Assess.* **3**(8).

42 Merelle ME, Nagelkerke AF, Lees CM and Dezateux C (2004) *Newborn Screening for Cystic Fibrosis (Cochrane Review).* The Cochrane Library, Issue 2. John Wiley and Sons, Chichester.

43 Stewart R and Oliver S (2004) *What is Known about Communication with Parents about Newborn Bloodspot Screening?* www.newbornscreening-bloodspot.org.uk/

44 West of Scotland Regional Genetics Service (2002) *Newborn Screening*; www.gla.ac.uk/medicalgenetics/nhs/biogeneonate.htm

45 David TJ (2004) Newborn screening for cystic fibrosis. *J R Soc Med.* **97**: 209–10.

46 Farrell MH and Farrell PM (2003) Newborn screening for cystic fibrosis: ensuring more good than harm. *J Pediatr.* **143**: 707–12.

47 Standing Medical Advisory Committee (1969) *Screening for the Detection of Congenital Dislocation of the Hip in Infants.* Department of Health and Social Security, London.

48 Jones D (1998) Neonatal detection of developmental dysplasia of the hip (DDH) (editorial). *J Bone Joint Surg.* **80-B**: 943–4.

49 Jones D, Dezateux CA, Danielsson LG, Paton RW and Clegg J (2000) Topics for debate: at the crossroads – neonatal detection of developmental dysplasia of the hip. *J Bone Joint Surg.* **82-B**: 260–64.

50 Standing Medical Advisory Committee and Standing Nursing and Midwifery Advisory Committee (1986) *Screening for the Detection of Congenital Dislocation of the Hip.* Department of Health and Social Security, London.

51 Dezateux C and Goodward S (1996) A national survey of screening for congenital dislocation of the hip. *Arch Dis Child.* **74**: 445–8.

52 Holen KH, Tegnander A and Bredland T (2002) Universal or selective screening of the neonatal hip. *J Bone Joint Surg.* **84-B**: 886–90.

53 Von Kries R, Ihme N, Oberle D *et al.* (2003) Effect of ultrasound screening on the rate of first operative procedures for developmental hip dysplasia in Germany. *Lancet.* **362**: 1883–7.

54 Marks DS, Clegg J and Al-Chalabi AN (1994) Routine ultrasound screening for neonatal hip instability: can it abolish late-presenting congenital dislocation of the hip? *J Bone Joint Surg.* **76-B**: 534–48.

55 Godward S and Dezateuz C on behalf of the MRC Working Group on Congenital Dislocation of the Hip (1998) Surgery for congenital dislocation of the hip in the UK as a measure of outcome of screening. *Lancet.* **351**: 1149–52.

56 Elbourne D, Dezateux C, Arthur R *et al.* on behalf of the UK Collaborative Hip Trial Group (2002) Ultrasonography in the diagnosis and management of developmental hip dysplasia (UK Hip Trial): clinical and economic results of a multicentre randomised controlled trial. *Lancet.* **360**: 2009–17.

57 Eastwood DM (2003) Neonatal hip screening. *Lancet.* **361**: 595–7.

58 Davis A, Bamford J *et al.* (1997) A critical review of neonatal hearing screening in the detection of congenital hearing screening impairment. *Health Technol Assess Rev.* **1**(10).

59 Newborn Hearing Screening Programme (NHSP); www.nhsp.info/

Chapter 5

Screening and surveillance in childhood and adolescence

The key to preventing many adult diseases lies in childhood when lifetime patterns of diet, exercise and moderation are most often set.*

Small children disturb your sleep, big children your life.†

Introduction

Screening and surveillance in childhood are important both in following up difficulties identified during the neonatal period and in diagnosing disorders for which effective treatment is available. This should be a seamless extension from antenatal and neonatal care, and it provides the opportunity to establish a basis for good health in later life with appropriate advice on healthy eating, home and road safety and immunisation. All reasonable steps should be taken at this early stage to promote good health and prevent illness.

Screening for older children and young people is another crucial area where there is scope for sensitive screening. Furthermore, this period of life is a time when formal contact with the health service is infrequent for most individuals. However, it is also a time when individuals are coping with profound physical and emotional changes and seeking their independence, but often lack the experience and judgement to use it wisely: 'The contrariness of adolescents is notorious: they are hypochondriacal yet mistrust doctors; they need support and collaboration from parents and teachers but go out of their way to make this difficult.'[1] This time of life has not become any easier in recent years – with an increase in the availability and usage of drugs and cheap alcohol, and a youth culture that encourages under-age and binge drinking and promiscuous sexual behaviour.

Childhood

There has been variation and some confusion in the use of the terms 'screening' and 'surveillance' in the context of childhood. For example, Bain[2] defined surveillance as a continuing process throughout childhood, and as part of the normal contact between the primary care team and the children on their list. Screening is a specific contact made by the team with an apparently healthy child in order to identify any mental or physical abnormalities. Bain cited the advantages of the process as the building of a positive relationship between the

---

* Hayman LL, Mahon MM and Turner JR (2003) *Health and Behavior in Childhood and Adolescence*. Springer Publishing Company, New York.
† Yiddish proverb.

parents and their child and primary care professionals, early identification of problems which can be treated or ameliorated, and improved immunisation rates. Disadvantages would include the use of limited resources of time and money for the routine examination of normal children, and differential attendance at clinics, with non-attendance being highest in the lower socio-economic groups who are at highest risk of illness.

The first Report of the Joint Working Group on Child Health Surveillance,* entitled *Health for All Children* and published in 1989,[3] defined surveillance broadly to cover assessment and monitoring of the physical, social and emotional health and development of all children, offering and arranging appropriate interventions when necessary, preventing disease by immunisation and other means, and health education.

In an independent review of child health surveillance, Butler[4] deplored the multiplicity of meanings given by different researchers to the term, but accepted that 'no set of definitions can be produced that will harmonise with the entire body of literature on preventive child care.'

In response to evolving professional thinking, the third edition of *Health for All Children*,[5] published in 1996, propounded the message that preventive health services for children should extend beyond the narrow remit of child health surveillance with its focus on the detection of abnormalities, and include efforts to prevent illness and promote good health. Following the suggestion of Butler, child health surveillance was re-defined as 'activities related to secondary prevention, that is, the detection of defects,' and was regarded as just one component of a child health promotion programme.

In practice, a rigid distinction between screening and surveillance in childhood is unrealistic. Routine surveillance of children in primary care can use screening as a specific tool for particular conditions, or in high-risk groups to try to prevent or treat illness.

The fourth edition of *Health for All Children*,[6] published in 2003, continued the move from a mainly disease-oriented model of screening for specific disorders to a greater emphasis on health promotion, primary prevention and active intervention for children at risk, whether for medical or social reasons. The editors state that the past decade of rising prosperity for many has been accompanied by increasing levels of violence, family breakdown, disaffection and alienation, and the gap between rich and poor has widened in the UK as it has elsewhere. These social changes must have an impact on children and their development.

The draft guidance on implementation of *Health for All Children* in Scotland in infancy and primary school is shown in Tables 5.1 to 5.4, and provides a useful summary on action to be taken at various stages.[7]

Despite the increasing emphasis on primary prevention, secondary prevention and screening for early detection of abnormalities remain important in terms of treatment and support of various kinds for affected children and their parents.

The Child Health Subgroup of the National Screening Committee now has a Child Health Screening Programme which aims to prevent or identify conditions that may impair development and accentuate inequalities.[8]

---

* This was a multi-disciplinary working party set up by the British Paediatric Association (now the Royal College of Paediatrics and Child Health) to review routine health checks for young children.

Table 5.1 Action recommended at 12–15 months

12–15 months	Comment
Action to be taken primarily by GP, practice or public health nurse	
Immunisation – MMR	Whoever is responsible for immunisation must be able to deal with questions about vaccines
Weight measurement	Whoever is responsible for weight measurement must be able to explain the weight chart
Health promotion	Discuss development, safety, nutrition, smoking, oral health, registration with a dentist, parenting skills, support networks and services, and any parental concerns

Table 5.2 Action recommended at 3–4 and 4–5 years

3–4 years	Comment
Action to be taken by lead professionals (could be public health nurse, GP, practice nurse or community paediatrician)	
Immunisation – PV, MMR and DTaP	Whoever is responsible for immunisation must be able to deal with questions about vaccines
Weight measurement	Whoever is responsible for weight measurement must be able to explain the weight chart
Health promotion	Discuss development, safety, nutrition, smoking, oral health, registration with a dentist, parenting skills, support networks and services, and any parental concerns
4–5 years	
Action to be taken by orthoptist	
Vision screen	Where preschool orthoptist vision screening cannot be implemented immediately, children should instead be screened on school entry. As a minimum, training and monitoring should be provided by an orthoptist

PV, pertussis; DTaP, diphtheria/tetanus/pertussis.

Table 5.3 Action recommended at entry to primary school

Entry to primary school	Comment
Action to be taken by school health service and community dental service	
Height	1990 nine-centile charts agreed as standard
Weight	
Record body mass index (for public health monitoring purposes only)	
Sweep test of hearing	Continue pending further review
Identify children who may not have received pre-school healthcare programme	
Identify any physical, developmental or emotional problems that have been missed, and initiate intervention	There is no evidence to justify a full physical examination or health review based on questionnaires or interviews on school entry
Check that preschool vision screening has been undertaken	If not, undertake on school entry
Ensure that all children have access to primary health and dental care	
Dental check at Primary 1 through the National Dental Inspection Programme	This identifies children at greatest risk of oral disease and is used to inform the school health plan
Oral health promotion	
Dentist registration and attendance	
Twice daily supervised brushing	
Reducing sugary food and drink consumption	

Table 5.4 Action recommended at Primary 7

Primary 7	Comment
Action to be taken by school health service and community dental service	
Dental health through National Dental Health Inspection Programme	This identifies children at greatest risk of oral disease and is used to inform the school health plan
Oral health promotion Dentist registration and attendance Twice daily supervised brushing Reducing sugary food and drink consumption	
Other health promotion activity to include smoking, nutrition, physical activity, substance use, sexual health, personal health, mental health and well-being	Development of an effective core programme of health promotion in schools is based on the roll-out of Health-Promoting Schools

Table 5.5 Conditions covered by the Child Health Screening Programme

Condition	Current NSC policy	Comment
Amblyopia and impaired vision	Other than those identified at neonatal screening, identification of visual defects under the age of 4 years should rely on parental concerns and professional awareness. Orthoptists should screen children in the 4–5 years age group with the aim of testing all children by the age of 5 years	Screening in 7-year-olds to be discontinued Position to be kept under review
Cryptorchidism	Part of neonatal screening Desirability of subsequent examinations under review	Update ongoing
Dental disease	Early contact with dentist to be encouraged. Dental screening at school should continue as required by law, but should be subject to formal review	Review ongoing
Developmental dysplasia of the hip (DDH)	Case finding and clinical approach. Children identified at neonatal screening to be kept under review. Parental observations and concerns are important	Would not meet criteria as a new programme, but ingrained in clinical practice. Training for examiners should be improved
Impaired growth	Height and weight to be measured around the time of school entry and the 0.4 cut-off for height should be used for initiation of referral	To be kept under review
Impaired hearing	Screening for hearing loss in school-age children should continue at present	Results of commissioned research awaited

The conditions included in the programme are summarised in Table 5.5. Those not considered suitable in view of the current state of knowledge are summarised in Table 5.6.

Physical examination

The school health service, established in 1908, introduced periodic medical examinations to detect previously unidentified diseases and abnormalities. The decline in many diseases and the availability of free universal access to healthcare since the inception of the NHS in 1948 have greatly reduced the likelihood that a child will start school with a previously undetected serious medical disorder.

Table 5.6 Conditions not considered suitable for screening with current state of knowledge

Condition	Current NSC policy	Comment
Autism	Not recommended on present evidence	To be kept under review
Developmental and behavioural problems	Screening for these complex conditions does not meet NSC criteria. Other approaches necessary to prevent and mitigate these problems and their effects	To be kept under review
Hyperlipidaemia	Cascade screening of relatives of patients with confirmed familial hyperlipidaemia	To be kept under review
Hypertension	Not recommended on present evidence	To be kept under review
Hypertrophic cardiomyopathy	Universal screening not recommended	To be kept under review
Iron-deficiency anaemia	Screening not recommended. Emphasis should be on primary prevention by providing good nutritional advice	To be kept under review
Lead poisoning	Not recommended	To be kept under review
Obesity	Not recommended on present evidence. Other approaches must be used to prevent and mitigate this problem and its effects	To be kept under review
Scoliosis	Not recommended	To be kept under review
Speech and language delay	Screening not recommended (HTA)	To be kept under review

HTA, Health Technology Assessment.

One would expect parents and the primary healthcare team to identify most children in need of attention (e.g. in terms of growth impairment, obesity or undescended testes), and it would be difficult to justify offering every apparently healthy child a full physical examination at school entry. Hall and Elliman recommend that the routine medical examination at school entry should be discontinued except as part of research studies.[6]

Nevertheless, there will be some children who miss out on healthcare (e.g. newly arrived refugees, deprived or homeless children), and a case can be made for some kind of health appraisal at the age of 5 years and the start of compulsory schooling for those who have missed out on earlier attention because of their lifestyle (e.g. travellers).

Hearing impairment

Permanent childhood hearing impairment (PCHI) can result from sensorineural or conductive hearing loss. Whatever the cause, it is important that it is identified early so that intervention can be started in order to minimise difficulties in language acquisition and social and educational development.

In 1997, Davis and colleagues[9] conducted a review of the literature and of current preschool hearing screening provision in the UK. They found that approximately 840 children are born each year with significant hearing impairment, and that services at that time would miss about 400 of these by 1½ years of age and about 200 by 3½ years.

Their survey highlighted a major problem along with poor information systems. They recommended that the NSC should urgently consider a national screening programme for congenital hearing impairment. They recommended a programme based on universal neonatal screening followed at 7 months by a targeted screen using the infant distraction test (mainly for those who had not had the neonatal screen) as the most equitable, responsive and cost-effective method.

As was discussed in Chapter 4, a universal neonatal screening programme for hearing impairment has now been agreed on the advice of the NSC, and is currently the subject of ongoing pilot studies before national roll-out.

Screening between the age of 1 year and school entry is not recommended either by the NSC[8] or by Hall and Elliman.[6] However, parents of preschool children should be asked routinely if they have any concerns about their child's hearing. Audiological assessment should be arranged for any child with markedly impaired language development, history of repeated middle-ear disease or behavioural problems.

The school entry 'sweep' test is still used throughout the UK and should be continued subject to research review. Very few children with significant hearing impairment will be identified at this late stage, but it may be useful in those newly arrived from overseas and those with a progressive hearing loss.

In 2001, Fortnum and colleagues[10] found that the prevalence of confirmed permanent childhood hearing impairment increases until the age of 9 years to a level higher than was previously estimated. If the current yield from screening is sustained, then for every ten children detected by neonatal screening, another five to nine children would show hearing impairment by the age of 9 years. These additional children would include some with congenital impairments who miss neonatal screening or pass the screening test despite their disability, some who acquire an impairment after the neonatal period, and others who show late-onset or progressive impairment. As Davis and colleagues[11] emphasise, there is a need to develop and implement more effective screening and case finding in school–age children (4–16 years) with acquired and late-onset impairments that may have a negative impact on their behaviour and educational achievement.

Russ[12] stresses the importance of evaluating neonatal hearing screening, and suggests that national databases should be established with core data on permanent childhood hearing impairment 'so long as this can be achieved in a way that maintains patient confidentiality and is acceptable to the community.'[12] This would certainly help to improve information systems and aid constructive research.

Further universal screening tests of hearing after school entry cannot be justified but, as in the preschool period, any child with learning, behavioural, speech or language difficulties should be audiologically assessed.

Visual impairment

A significant number of serious visual disorders are likely to be found at the routine neonatal examination, and the available evidence suggests that formal visual screening of every infant in the first year of life is not justified.

There are difficulties in testing the vision of preschool children, and testing before the age of 4 years appears to produce too many unreliable results to make it a satisfactory screening procedure. However, waiting until school entry may result in a less satisfactory outcome in terms of treatment of amblyopia.

Snowdon and Stewart-Brown[13] undertook a systematic review of the effectiveness of preschool vision screening in relation to three target conditions, namely amblyopia, refractive errors, and squints that are not cosmetically obvious. They found a lack of good-quality research into the natural history of the conditions, the disabilities that they cause and the efficacy of treatment. This evidence is essential to justify a screening programme for a non-fatal condition in the absence of rigorous controlled trials. An invitation to preschool vision screening carries the implicit assumption that screening will benefit the child and, on this basis, the ethical justification for such screening is weak.

Williams and colleagues,[14] in a study designed to assess the effectiveness of early treatment for amblyopia in 3490 children, compared intensive orthoptic screening at 8, 12, 18, 25, 31 and 37 months (intensive group) with orthoptic screening at 37 months only (control group). They found that early treatment is more effective in reducing the severity of the problem than later treatment, supporting the principle of preschool vision screening. An important question for further research is whether programmes in routine practice could deliver the same benefits as the intensive programme without the need for repeated testing, which would be very costly.

Rahi and Dezateux[15–17] have drawn attention to the fact that despite the neonatal examination, a substantial proportion of children with congenital and infantile cataract are not being diagnosed. They call for strategies to achieve better detection through screening and surveillance. Their proposals for screening and surveillance for vision and ophthalmic disorders in childhood are summarised in Table 5.7.

Rahi and Dezateux also call for further research on the effects of age at the start of treatment for amblyopia on outcome, and on whether a childhood screening programme results in a meaningful and sustained reduction in the prevalence of the condition in adolescence and early adulthood.

Clarke and colleagues,[18] in a study of 177 children aged 3–5 years in eight UK eye departments, found that children with a moderate loss of acuity showed a clear-cut response to treatment, in contrast to those with mild acuity loss who received little benefit. Delay in treatment until the age of 5 years did not appear to influence effectiveness. They suggest that low-level impairment is still commonly treated in routine clinical practice but that this may not be justified.

Further research in this area is clearly needed. Detection and treatment of amblyopia are beneficial in at least some children, and the focus should now be on optimising screening strategies to obtain the best results.[19]

Table 5.7 UK proposals for screening and surveillance for vision and ophthalmic disorders in childhood

Target population	Recommendation
Neonatal period and early infancy Very-low-birthweight and premature babies	Specialist ophthalmic examination to detect retinopathy of prematurity
All newborns and 6- to 8-week-old infants	Newborn and 6–8 week examination to detect media opacities (particularly congenital cataract) and eye anomalies
Infancy to primary school age (4 years and under)	Discontinue routine screening examinations for strabismus and amblyopia by orthoptists and health visitors
Primary school age (all 4- to 5-year-olds)	Introduce primary screening by orthoptists for strabismus and amblyopia
Secondary school age (11 years and over)	Insufficient evidence to recommend either discontinuation of existing or introduction of new vision screening programmes for refractive errors

Source: Rahi and Dezateux.[17] Reproduced with kind permission of the authors and Elsevier.

Elliman and colleagues[20] emphasise that training and supervision of those performing neonatal examination of the eyes must be improved. They also point out that the resource implications of orthoptist screening of all children by the age of 5 years need to be examined in more detail. And although the evidence in favour of all other vision testing in school-age children is weak, they suggest that existing screening programmes should continue for the time being.

There is evidence that socially disadvantaged adults are less likely to have their eyes tested and more likely to have treatable but undiagnosed eye problems. If this is also found to be true of children, a further universal screening test may be required to offer more equitable care, although further research is needed. There is also a need for further research into screening for defects of colour vision and the relationship between vision and dyslexia. Parental observations and concerns should be taken seriously and investigated, and any child with learning difficulties or other school problems should have their vision checked.

The gold standard would seem to be the examination by orthoptists of all children between the ages of 4 and 5 years. This is the current policy.

Developmental screening

There is currently no evidence to support population screening for developmental delay in general.[20]

Law and colleagues[21] undertook a systematic review of research into the value of screening and intervention for speech and language delays in children up to the age of 7 years. They found insufficient evidence to merit the introduction of universal screening, but suggested that more attention should be paid to the role of parents in identifying children with speech and language delays, and to providing information and support for them in less formal ways.

At present there is no satisfactory screening test for autism.[22]

A retrospective study looking at the effectiveness of developmental screening in identifying learning disabilities in early childhood found that many children experienced delay in referral to the appropriate remedial services.[23] In many cases the interval between initial parental identification and referral was more than 12 months. Reasons for delay in seeking specialist care included late identification of some children with problems, assessment and referral by professionals working individually rather than as a multi-disciplinary team, and a lack of awareness of the importance of early intervention.

Developmental abnormalities or delays of whatever kind in childhood are obviously of great concern to parents, who are often likely to be the first to identify possible problems. Although at present there is no evidence to support a universal screening approach, this should be kept under research review, and parental anxieties should be taken seriously and dealt with initially in the primary care/community setting with referral as appropriate. In some cases, training of staff may be necessary to ensure the development of the skills necessary to identify need for referral.

Dental screening

The Child Health Subgroup of the NSC produced a report on dental disease in December 2003.[8] The report noted that dental screening has to be provided for schoolchildren with at least three separate screens, the first on school entry. It is also policy to recommend parents to register their children with a dentist before they are 2 years of age, and to take them for regular checks thereafter. Only 22% of parents take this advice and, unsurprisingly, this is strongly related to social class. There is also a problem with the scarcity of NHS dentists in some areas of the country.

Research on various aspects of dental screening has been commissioned, and the results should help to clarify policy. For the moment, school dental screening should continue but should undergo formal review. This is another area where efforts need to be made to reduce existing inequalities whereby the most deprived children are the least likely to receive dental attention.

Developmental dysplasia and congenital dislocation of the hip

The Child Health Screening Programme includes recommendation of a case-finding approach to screening hips at this stage to review children identified by neonatal screening and diagnose any who have been missed earlier. Again parental observations and concerns about gait or late walking should be taken seriously, and training for those performing the clinical examination should be improved with high-quality ultrasound to check on clinical findings where necessary. As was discussed in Chapter 4, universal screening for CDH in the neonatal period was introduced almost 40 years ago. However, despite this there remain wide variations in practice and quality between centres in different parts of the country[24] and there is a risk of over-diagnosis and over-treatment.[25]

Eastwood's conclusion – that there is an urgent need to define exactly what to screen for and how to treat – applies as much in childhood as in the neonatal period where universal screening takes place.[26]

Conclusion

Our recommendations on screening in childhood are summarised in Table 5.8.

Childhood is the time to build on the care given in the antenatal and neonatal periods that should have identified any major problems and instigated treatment where appropriate. Vigilance in finding any abnormalities not previously detected is important, but the vast majority of children are healthy and the focus should be on laying good foundations for maintenance of that health in the future. The growing problem of childhood obesity is not at present a candidate for screening, although advice on weight control, exercise and healthy eating should be available in primary care and in school. Since weight/height measurements are taken regularly at various ages by GPs and in schools, action should be taken on the results to try to improve the diet of children and encourage their participation in games and exercise, rather than submitting them to a 'screening' test.

The more deprived and disadvantaged children and those recently arrived from abroad as refugees or asylum seekers may have missed out on earlier medical and

Table 5.8 Our recommendations for screening in childhood

Condition	Comment
Hearing impairment	Follow-up on neonatal programme where indicated
	School entry 'sweep' test to continue for the time being
	Case finding to identify late-onset or progressive impairment
	Investigation of any children with educational or behavioural problems
Amblyopia and impaired vision	Orthoptist screening in 4- to 5-year-olds as per NSC policy
	Attention to be paid to children who miss this test for any reason
Dental disease	School dental screening mandatory and should continue but be kept under research review
	Early contact with dentists to be encouraged
	Problems include shortage of NHS dentists and lack of parental compliance, especially among more deprived families
CHD/DDH	Children identified by neonatal screening to be reviewed
	Parental observations and concerns to be investigated
Deprived, disadvantaged or socially isolated children	Need to identify such children and instigate screening/case finding where relevant

dental checks, and strenuous efforts should be made to identify them and make sure that any omissions or inequities are minimised.

Adolescence

The boundaries between childhood and adolescence are blurring, with many children appearing to mature earlier, physically if not emotionally. In this chapter we shall regard adolescence as the period from the start of secondary school until the early twenties.

This is a difficult period of adjustment towards adulthood and one that is poorly understood, partly because of the difficulties of communication. Reviewing a recent book on difficult consultations with teenagers, MacAuley[27] acknowledges that 'talking to a different generation can be like communicating with aliens ... it is as difficult for us to understand adolescents as it is for them to understand us.'

The focus of screening and surveillance at this sensitive stage should take account of what adolescents and young adults themselves feel they require and how it can be most effectively provided.

Health for All Children[5] cites a survey by the Home Office, which found that young people listed the following as their main needs:

- accessible confidential health services
- greater involvement of young people in planning services
- health education that reflects their experiences, especially with regard to drugs and alcohol
- specialised advice centres for those with drug problems.

Young people acquire attitudes to healthcare and obtain much of their information in this area from their peer group. This needs to be acknowledged when planning screening and other health-related services for this age group.

The fourth report of a large, ongoing World Health Organization-funded survey of health behaviour in teenagers across Europe and North America has shown widespread differences between boys and girls with regard to health behaviours and attitudes, which need to be better understood.[28]

Many issues are relevant, including stress, depression, abuse, bullying and violence, contraception, sexual health and substance misuse. There is a need for confidential advice, support and if necessary intervention to be available, and this can be provided by health professionals in a number of ways. Teachers also have a role to play in identifying potential problems. Older children and adolescents may prefer a more discreet approach with drop-in clinics away from school premises.

The official guidance on a programme for health screening and surveillance in secondary school is summarised in Table 5.9.[29]

This programme, if carried out and adhered to assiduously, should result in a healthy population of young people, but it is non-specific and its application will vary widely from school to school. Unfortunately, those most at risk – due, for example, to deprivation, refugee or homeless status – will be less likely to submit to this type of surveillance. On a purely practical level, one wonders how many perfectly conscientious parents will achieve 'twice daily supervised toothbrushing' with a prickly mid-teenager.

Table 5.9 Core programme for health screening and surveillance in secondary school

---

Action to be taken by school health service and community dental service

Age 10–14 years BCG immunisation

In areas where vision is checked at 11 years, this should continue pending review by the NSC. Where it is not already being checked, it should not be introduced

Age 13–18 years – poliovirus (PV) and (Td) immunisation

Dental check at S3 through National Dental Inspection Programme

Oral health promotion

    Dentist registration and attendance

    Twice daily supervised brushing

    Reducing intake of sugary food and drink

Other health promotion activity

    Smoking

    Sexual health

    Nutrition

    Personal safety

    Physical activity

    Mental health and well-being

    Substance misuse

Dental checks

National Dental Inspection Programme identifies children at greatest risk of oral disease and is used to inform the school health plan

Health promotion

Development of an effective core programme of health promotion in schools is premised on the roll-out of Health-Promoting Schools

---

Health education and promotion

Health promotion can be a potent tool in this arena, but if it is to have any impact it must be effectively pitched for its market. Young people are notoriously careless of their own health: 'They cope with the impact of mortality by pretending they are immortal, and challenge fate by jaywalking across busy roads, drinking and taking drugs. What matters is now, today. Not what might happen tomorrow.'[30]

For example, people who smoke, unless they are unable to read the messages on cigarette packets, cannot be unaware of the risks they are running. The Health Education Board for Scotland had considerable success with a campaign featuring a fictitious girl band – Stinx – and a song that debunked the spuriously fashionable and glamorous image of smoking.[31] There was positive feedback from young people across Scotland, and the resulting CD reached the singles charts in Scotland and in the UK. However, efforts to ban tobacco advertising in any form and end smoking in public places continue to be strongly opposed both by those who perceive this as an infringement of their freedom of choice and, of course, by the tobacco manufacturers.

Drug and alcohol misuse, serious as their effects are, are not areas where screening is appropriate. The main weapon again has to be health promotion, with treatment and support where it is needed. Scenes of binge drinking and violence are now commonplace in many city centres throughout the UK on Friday and Saturday nights. The burden that this places on police, hospital and prison services must be huge, in terms of both time and money. Restriction of 'happy hours' is now being implemented in some areas in an effort to reduce the problem. However, in the light of all this, the political decision to liberalise pub opening times seems a curious one.

Injury and suicide prevention is also a priority in this age group, and there is a need for research into screening for risk.

Scoliosis

Reviewing the evidence on scoliosis, the National Screening Committee concluded that screening cannot be recommended at the present time. This will be kept under review.

The difficulties here include over-diagnosis and doubts about the efficacy of the available treatment for those identified as being affected. As Berwick pointed out almost 20 years ago:

> To make rational policy we at least need better data on the psychological morbidity for false positives, the effectiveness of treatment of moderate curves, the worth of exercises and the marginal contributions of screening compared with spontaneous detection rates. Without such data, the hunt is as likely to be leading us into the swamp as towards our quarry.[32]

The difficulties identified by Berwick remain relevant today, and any serious problems of this nature seem likely to be identified by the affected individuals themselves, their parents or their general practitioners, and dealt with accordingly.

Sexual health

Contraception

The UK has the highest rate of teenage births in Western Europe, six times the rate in Holland. This has obvious health and social repercussions for the young people involved, their children and society in general. The Government has launched a national campaign to halve the rate of conception among under-18-year-olds by 2010, and a cross-departmental ministerial task force has been established, chaired by the Minister for Public Health, with a Department of Health unit overseeing implementation.

Clearly, there is a need for action and for more effective health education and confidential contraceptive advice in this area. Recent high-profile cases involving parents who were outraged when they were not informed, for example, of a daughter's pregnancy, have tended to obscure rather than reveal the facts. Each case must be judged on its own merits, and there may well be family tensions and circumstances of which the media are unaware that make the teenager's request for confidentiality paramount. However, parents' rights must also be taken into account, as in most cases they are best placed to provide the guidance and support necessary, based on a lifetime's knowledge of their own child.

In any case, the law on under-age contraception is clear.[33] Under-16-year-olds:

- have a right to confidentiality of their discussions with medical practitioners
- should not fear being reported to their parents just for consulting a doctor or nurse
- can obtain contraceptive treatment without parental consent if certain conditions are met.

In 1989 the US Preventive Services Task Force[34] recommended that clinicians should obtain a detailed sexual history from all adolescent patients: 'Empathy, confidentiality and a non-judgemental supportive attitude were stressed.'

The Canadian Task Force on the Periodic Health Examination echoed this view in 1993, concluding that there is fair evidence that physicians can reduce the toll of unwanted pregnancy 'by provision of education and contraception services, by involving pubertal patients and, where appropriate, their parents in early open discussion of sexual development, prevention of sexually transmitted diseases, and prevention of unwanted pregnancies.'[35]

This is difficult territory, in which good health education and access to confidential and supportive advice in an acceptable setting, rather than screening and surveillance, are what is required. One existing model of such practice is the Sandyford Initiative in Glasgow, where young people can access advice and support in a drop-in centre and via a website.[36]

Chlamydia

Chlamydia trachomatis infection is the UK's most common curable sexually transmitted bacterial infection. It is often asymptomatic or produces only mild, non-specific signs in both men and women. In women, the infection can lead to life-threatening ectopic pregnancies, pelvic inflammatory disease and infertility.

Almost 70 000 cases of chlamydia were diagnosed in clinics in 2001, representing an increase of 10% on the previous year. This is therefore an issue of major and growing concern in relation to the health of young people.[37]

In Scotland, a National Sexual Health Demonstration Project – *Healthy Respect* – was launched in late October 2000 with the aim of testing different interventions and approaches to improving the sexual health of young people.[38] This included a project designed to explore opportunities for screening for chlamydia in non-medical settings.

In April 2001, a report on a systematic review of screening for chlamydial infection was published by the US Agency for Healthcare Research and Quality.[39] It concluded that chlamydia infection presents an ideal screening opportunity. Adolescents and young adults have the highest prevalence rates, and the infection is usually symptomless and therefore undetected in the absence of screening. It is easily diagnosed by non-invasive urine tests, and can be effectively treated with antibiotics. The most difficult aspect of screening is determining exactly who and how frequently to screen, and further research is needed in this area.

As background to this, a major study was started in the UK in 2001 involving researchers at the universities of Bristol and Birmingham, the Public Health Laboratory Service and local GPs in the Midlands area.[40]

Moens and colleagues[41] conducted a cross-sectional study of chlamydia infection in an inner-city contraceptive and psychotherapy service for young people aged 12–21 years. They offered testing by urine sample to all young people using the contraceptive service who had not already been screened.

They found that screening in this way was acceptable to young women, who found it less stigmatising than having to attend a sexual health clinic, and that the non-invasive urine test was more acceptable than vaginal examination and swabs.

Moens and colleagues emphasise the key role of reception staff, who need to be well trained in communicating sensitive information and in ensuring that individuals who are infected do return for treatment. They had less success in reaching male partners of those who were found to be positive, and this aspect needs further study.

Tong and colleagues[42] stressed the need for microbiological input when screening for chlamydia, in order to avoid inappropriate labelling of individuals, unnecessary partner notification and over-treatment.

The National Screening Committee has commissioned a programme of opportunistic screening for young people of both sexes under the age of 25 years who access the sexual health services. The phased implementation of the National Chlamydia Screening Programme began in 2002 after the successful pilot studies in Bristol and Birmingham. A total of 26 local chlamydia screening programmes have already been implemented in two phases, with a third phase due to be launched shortly. The objective is to achieve national coverage by 2008 in a way that will not swamp the health service.

Conclusion

The only opportunistic screening programme that we would consider appropriate in adolescence is the already established and phased programme for chlamydia (*see* Table 5.10).

> The great paradox of adolescence is that between the great highs of screaming and singing through the streets and feeling more independent are the great lows: deep loneliness, boredom and that terrifying new awareness of how small and alone we are in the world. As the mind and body mature, the full reality of human frailty becomes apparent.[30]

We must endeavour to understand this stage of life better. The most constructive approach is opportunistic case finding in primary and community care, with sensitive and confidential advice, support and health education provided in a way and in a setting that is acceptable and helpful to young people to enable them more successfully to bridge the difficult gap between childhood and maturity.

Table 5.10 Our recommendation for screening in adolescence and early adulthood

Condition	Comment
Chlamydia	Phased implementation of opportunistic screening of those aged 25 years or under who access sexual health services

References

1 Spicer RF (1990) Adolescents. In: WW Holland, R Detels and EG Knox (eds) *Oxford Textbook of Public Health* (2e). *Volume 3, Section D. Needs of special client groups.* Oxford University Press, Oxford.

2 Bain J (1989) Developmental screening for pre-school children: is it worthwhile? *J R Coll Gen Pract.* **39**: 133–7.

3 Hall DMB (ed.) (1989) *Health for All Children: a programme of child health surveillance. Report of the Joint Working Party on Child Health Surveillance.* Oxford University Press, Oxford.

4 Butler JR (1989) *Child Health Surveillance in Primary Care: a critical review.* HMSO, London.

5 Hall D (ed.) (1996) *Health for All Children* (3e). Oxford University Press, Oxford.

6 Hall DMB and Elliman D (eds) (2003) *Health for All Children* (4e). Oxford University Press, Oxford.

7 www.scotland.gov.uk/consultations/health/hfac-06.asp

8 www.nelh.nhs.uk/screening/child

9 Davis A, Bamford J, Wilson I, Ramkalawan T, Forshaw M and Wright S (1991) A critical review of the role of neonatal hearing screening in the detection of childhood hearing impairment. *Health Technol Assess.* **1**(10).

10 Fortnum HM, Summerfield AQ, Marshall DH, Davis AC and Bamford JM (2001) Prevalence of permanent childhood hearing impairment in the United Kingdom and implications for universal neonatal hearing screening: questionnaire-based ascertainment study. *BMJ.* **323**: 536–40.

11 Davis A, Yoshinaga-Itano C and Hind S (2001) Universal newborn hearing screening: implications for coordinating and developing services for deaf and hearing-impaired children (commentary). *BMJ.* **323**: 540.

12 Russ S (2001) Measuring the prevalence of permanent childhood hearing impairment (editorial). *BMJ.* **323**: 525–6.

13 Snowdon SK and Stewart-Brown SL (1997) Preschool vision screening. *Health Technol Assess.* **1**(8).

14 Williams C, Northstone K, Harrad RA, Sparrow JM and Harvey I for the ALSPAC Study Team (2002) Amblyopia treatment outcomes after screening before or at age 3 years: follow-up from randomised trial. *BMJ.* **324**: 1549–51.

15 Rahi JS and Dezateux C (1999) National cross-sectional study of detection of congenital and infantile cataract in the UK: role of childhood screening and surveillance. *BMJ.* **318**: 362–5.

16 Rahi JS and Dezateux C for the British Congenital Cataract Interest Group (2001) Measuring and interpreting the incidence of congenital ocular anomalies: lessons from a National Study of Congenital Cataract in the UK. *Invest Ophthalmol Vis Sci.* **42**: 1444–8.

17 Rahi JS and Dezateux C (2002) Improving the detection of childhood visual problems and eye disorders. *Lancet.* **359**: 1083–4.

18 Clarke MP, Wright CM, Hrisos S, Anderson JD, Henderson J and Richardson SR (2003) Randomised controlled trial of unilateral visual impairment detected at preschool vision screening. *BMJ.* **327**: 1251–4.

19 Dutton GN and Cleary M (2003) Should we be screening for and treating amblyopia? (editorial). *BMJ.* **327**: 1242–3.

20 Elliman DAC, Dezateux C and Bedford HE (2002) Newborn and childhood screening programmes: criteria, evidence and current policy. *Arch Dis Child.* **87**: 6–9.

21 Law J, Boyle J, Harris F *et al.* (1998) Screening for speech and language delay: a systematic review of the literature. *Health Technol Assess.* **2**: 1–184.

22 Baron-Cohen S, Wheelwright S, Cox A *et al.* (2000) Early identification of autism by the Checklist for Autism in Toddlers (CHAT). *J R Soc Med.* **93**: 521–5.

23 Nuallain S and Flanagan O (2001) A study looking at the effectiveness of developmental screening in identifying learning disabilities in early childhood. *Ir Med J.* **94**. Online article.

24 Godward S and Dezateux C on behalf of the MRC Working Group on Congenital Dislocation of the Hip (1998) Surgery for congenital dislocation of the hip in the UK as a measure of outcome of screening. *Lancet.* **351**: 1149–52.

25 Jahn A and Razum O (2003) Neonatal hip screening. *Lancet.* **361**: 1659.

26 Eastwood DM (2003) Neonatal hip screening. *Lancet.* **361**: 595–7.

27 MacAuley D (2004) Book review of *Difficult Consultations with Adolescents. BMJ.* **328**: 1443.

28 Young People's Health in Context: health behaviour in school-aged children; www.euro.who.int

29 www.scotland.gov.uk/consultations/health/hfac-06.asp

30 Figes K (2004) *The Terrible Teens: what every parent needs to know.* Penguin, Harmondsworth.

31 Tannahill A (2003) Promoting health in Scotland. In: K Wood and D Carter (eds) *Scotland's Health and Health Services.* The Nuffield Trust, London.

32 Berwick DM (1985) Scoliosis screening: a pause in the chase. *Am J Public Health.* **75**: 1373–4.

33 www.healthforallchildren.co.uk

34 US Preventive Services Task Force (1989) *Guide to Clinical Preventive Services: an assessment of 169 interventions.* Williams and Wilkins, Baltimore, MD.

35 Feldman W, Martell A and Dingle JL (1993) *Prevention of Unintended Pregnancy and Sexually Transmitted Diseases in Adolescents.* Canadian Task Force on the Periodic Health Examination, Ottawa.

36 www.sandyford.org.

37 Chlamydia Screening Studies (ClaSS); www.chlamydia.ac.uk

38 www.healthy.respect.com

39 Nelson H, Saha S and Helfand M (2001) *Screening for Chlamydial Infection. A systematic evidence review.* AHRQ Publication No. 01-S003. Agency for Healthcare Research and Quality, Rockville, MD.

40 www.nelh.nhs.uk/screening/

41 Moens V, Baruch G and Fearon P (2003) Opportunistic screening for chlamydia as a community-based contraceptive service for young people. *BMJ.* **326**: 1252–5.

42 Tong CYW, Dunn H and Lewis DA (2003) Microbiological input is essential in chlamydia screening programmes (letter). *BMJ.* **327**: 290.

Chapter 6

Screening in adults

Medicine has no mandate to be meddlesome in the lives of those who do not need it.*

Introduction

Screening in adults is potentially big business. Private healthcare providers offer total Well Woman and Well Man screening programmes, and many pharmacies are now offering tests for diabetes and selling personal blood pressure and cholesterol monitors for use at home. Private screening organisations offer a variety of screening tests for a range of conditions, including osteoporosis, *Helicobacter pylori* and prostate cancer, from mobile units around the country, often parked in supermarket car parks. Media interest in health is insatiable. Most newspapers now have Health and Lifestyle sections with information on 'new' treatments and advice from health professionals on how to cope with various conditions and how to enhance physical and emotional well-being. Television programmes include endless 'in-depth' analyses of diseases as well as personal stories of the lives of patients suffering from some affliction.

Fitzpatrick suggests that health has become a new religion and illustrates how many terms now link health with daily life and permeate our thinking – healthy eating, exercise for health, sexual health, healthy lifestyles, and so on.[1] Traditionally, general practice was a demand-led service whereby individuals went to seek diagnosis and treatment for a specific complaint. However, over the past 10 years the emphasis has moved towards a more proactive approach on the part of both doctors and patients. Specific patient groups are invited for health and screening checks, and advantage is taken of routine consultations to provide advice on issues such as smoking and drinking, diet and exercise. Health-conscious patients request tests for conditions for which there is no evidence of screening benefit.

Fitzpatrick further suggests that 'instead of serving their patients' needs, GPs now serve the demands of government policy – and the dictates of government-imposed health promotion performance targets.'[1]

Adults are arguably more vulnerable to over-zealous screening practices than those at earlier stages of the life cycle. For the most part, babies, infants, children and adolescents undergo screening procedures within a framework designed to identify treatable conditions or to correct impairments in function in order to enable them to realise their full potential. Young adults, with the obvious exception of those in the processes of pregnancy and childbirth, tend to have low health service usage.

However, as life wears on, individuals – if they read, watch television or listen

---

* Skrabanek P (1994) *The Death of Humane Medicine*. Social Affairs Unit, London.

to the radio at all – can hardly fail to be made aware of the various health problems and diseases that may be lying in wait for them. Of course, it is of benefit if potential conditions can be identified early and treated, or at least alleviated. However, society must beware of turning health into an obsession and must resist both the increasing medicalisation of life and the growing politicisation of medicine. Above all we must make sure that before any further national screening programme is introduced, the long-established screening criteria are satisfied and the evidence base exists.

The National Screening Committee's position on screening in adults is summarised in Table 6.1.[2]

The main current contenders for screening in adults are various forms of cancer and cardiovascular disease allied to stroke, abdominal aortic aneurysm and diabetes, the leading causes of morbidity and mortality in both men and women. We shall also consider briefly a number of other diseases of middle age, as well as occupational screening.

Cancer

Cancer is the second largest cause of mortality in the UK and is responsible for a quarter of all deaths.[3] It is also a significant cause of morbidity, with 280 000 new cases diagnosed each year in England and Wales alone. It has been estimated that one in three individuals will develop some form of cancer during their lifetime, and the disease thus has substantial resource implications for the NHS.

Breast cancer

Breast cancer is now the largest cause of death in women under 65 years of age, and it kills around 15 000 women a year in the UK. The current position is that women aged between 50 and 70 years on population registers are invited for screening by mammography every three years through the National Breast Cancer Screening Programme. Women over the age of 70 years can be screened on request.

Two major studies of screening programmes in the USA[4] and in Sweden[5] during the 1980s found that around 30% of breast cancer deaths could be prevented by early detection of tumours and treatment. A follow-up study in Sweden reported an increasing fall in the number of deaths in those screened.[6] This led to enormous pressure from politicians, women's organisations, cancer charities and sections of the medical profession itself within the UK for a national screening programme. The report of a Working Group, chaired by Sir Patrick Forrest and published in 1987, concluded that there was a convincing clinical case for screening women aged 50–64 years.[7] The national programme began in 1988 and achieved national coverage in 1990.

Screening for breast cancer has generated more discussion than any other single screening procedure, and opinions on its value continue to vary. There are many who, like Hann,[8] consider that the decision to embark on a national screening programme was based on political rather than medical considerations, and question the whole rationale of the service. Others direct their criticisms to

Table 6.1 The National Screening Committee's recommendations for and against screening in adults*

Condition	Current policy	Comment
Abdominal aortic aneurysm	A case can be made for screening	Under review. Implementation being discussed
Alcohol problems	No evidence to support systematic screening	To be kept under review
Anal cancer	Population-based screening not supported by present evidence	Under review
Bladder cancer	Occupational screening for high-risk groups under consideration	To be kept under review
Breast cancer	National programme – women aged 50–70 years invited for mammography every 3 years. Women over 70 years screened on request	To be kept under review
Cervical cancer	National programme – women aged 25–64 years every 3–5 years depending on age	To be kept under review Programme converting to liquid-based cytology (LBC) over the next 5 years following pilot studies
Colorectal cancer	A working group has been set up to plan the introduction of screening	To be kept under review
Coronary heart disease	Diabetic, Heart Disease and Stroke Prevention Project being piloted in nine inner-city primary care trusts	To be kept under review
Depression	Population screening not recommended	To be kept under review
Diabetes	See entry for coronary heart disease	To be kept under review
Diabetic retinopathy	National screening programme for sight-threatening diabetic retinopathy is being rolled out across the UK	To be kept under review
Domestic violence	Screening not recommended. Further work ongoing	To be kept under review
Glaucoma	No action to be taken at present because of scale of work needed to achieve diabetic retinopathy targets	To be kept under review

Table continued overleaf

Table 6.1 (*continued*)

Condition	Current policy	Comment
Haemochromatosis	Review of evidence does not support screening	To be kept under review
Hepatitis C	Screening not recommended HTA evidence suggests that testing injecting drug users is cost-effective, but this is good clinical practice rather than screening	To be kept under review
Lung cancer	Current evidence does not support screening	To be kept under review
Oral cancer	Routine screening is not recommended	To be kept under review
Osteoporosis	Review of current evidence does not support screening	To be kept under review
Ovarian cancer	Routine screening is not recommended	To be kept under review
Prostate cancer	On the basis of two recent systematic reviews of the evidence, screening should not be introduced as a national programme	Because of the high level of demand for PSA testing, a Prostate Cancer Risk Management Programme has been introduced. Ongoing review
Renal disease	Population screening not recommended except as part of a peer-reviewed and ethically approved research project	To be kept under review
Stomach cancer	More research information required on screening for both gastric cancer and *Helicobacter pylori*	To be kept under review
Stroke	See entry for coronary heart disease	To be kept under review
Testicular cancer	No policy guidance	To be kept under review
Thrombophilia	No current evidence to support screening	To be kept under review
Thyroid disease	No screening except in the context of peer-reviewed and ethically approved research	To be kept under review

* Chlamydia is covered in Chapter 4 and Alzheimer's disease is covered in Chapter 7.
PSA, prostate-specific antigen.

service standards and coverage, which has varied between regions over the period 1991–2002 as shown in Table 6.2.

In England as a whole there has been a slight increase in coverage, from 71% to 75.6% over the 11-year period. There has been remarkable consistency in range between the worst and the best regions – around 15–20%. The worst regions were in London, particularly the North Thames Regions. The best regions were in the north, namely Trent, Northern and Yorkshire. In Wales, overall coverage was slightly lower and varied between 65% and 70% over the same time period.[9] In Scotland, approximately 152 000 women are invited for breast screening each year in one of six regional screening centres or 13 associated mobile screening units used in rural or inner-city areas, and around 74% of these women accept the invitation. The Scottish Breast Screening Programme detects around 3000 breast cancers per year.[10]

Proponents of screening believe that the programme is good both in principle and in practice, but still needs to be improved and extended.

There can be little doubt that mortality from breast cancer has fallen since the introduction of screening. Tabar and colleagues,[11] in a 20-year follow-up of the Swedish screening study, concluded that 'taking account of potential biases, changes in clinical practice and changes in the incidence of breast cancer,' mammographic screening is contributing to substantial reductions in breast cancer mortality in the two counties involved in the study. In 2002, Nystrom and colleagues[12] published an updated overview of the Swedish randomised trials and concluded that the advantageous effect of screening on breast cancer mortality persists after long-term follow-up, and that recent criticism of the trials is scientifically unfounded.

Blanks and colleagues[13] conducted an age cohort study to assess the impact of the national screening programme on mortality in women aged 55–59 over the period 1990–98. They concluded that by 1998 both screening and other factors,

Table 6.2 Coverage of breast cancer screening in England during the period 1991–2002*

Years	Worst region (%)	Best region (%)	Whole country(%)
1991–92	61	81	71
1992–93	61	79	72
1993–94	62	79	72
1994–95	68	84	77
1995–96	68	84	76
1996–97	65	82	75.5
1997–98	66	81	75.4
1998–99	65	81	76.2
1999–2000	62	81	75.6
2000–01	62	81	75.3
2001–02	63	82	75.6

* *Note:* some area boundaries have changed during this time period.

including improvements in treatment, had resulted in a substantial reduction in mortality from the disease, and they predicted further reductions, particularly for women aged 55–69 years, over the next 10 years.

However, many workers contend that the reduction in mortality cannot be attributed solely, or indeed mainly, to screening.

Botha and colleagues[14] examined long-term trends in the incidence of and mortality from breast cancer by age group in 16 European countries, and their relationship to the introduction of mammographic screening programmes in six of these countries. They suggest that the declines in mortality which have emerged since the late 1980s may be related in part to earlier detection by screening, but they point out that the declining trends started well before screening was introduced and occurred in non-screened age groups and in several countries without national screening programmes.

These researchers contend that improved care of patients with breast cancer either through new, more effective treatment, such as tamoxifen, or because of better access to care is the major determinant in countries without screening, and is also an important determinant in countries with screening programmes.

They conclude:

> While the beneficial effects of the widespread introduction of screening will continue to accrue for several years, it is clear that improvements in the management of women with breast cancer have had an important effect, and the development of high-quality care deserves our continued attention.[14]

In 2001, Olsen and Gøtzsche, writing in the *Lancet*, published a Cochrane Review on Screening for Breast Cancer with mammography, in which they criticised the studies that informed the decision to implement screening.[15] They suggested that 'the current available reliable evidence does not show a survival benefit of mass screening for breast cancer.'

Olsen and Gøtzsche drew attention to the problems of over-diagnosis and over-treatment, and pointed out that since most invasive cancers grow slowly, many might never manifest themselves in the absence of screening and become disease before the women died from other causes.

Baum,[16] one of the original pioneers of the national screening programme, also presented an eloquent case against mammographic screening.

Freedman and colleagues,[17] in a qualitative review of the evidence, countered these negative views in strong terms and defended the various studies and their findings. They concluded that the prior consensus in favour of screening by mammography was correct, and that there is good evidence from clinical trials that screening reduces the death rate from breast cancer.

The 2002 Annual Review of the Breast Screening Programme[18] acknowledged the controversy, and quoted the conclusion of the International Agency for Research on Cancer (IARC) of the World Health Organization that 'regular mammographic screening of women between 50 and 69 will save the lives of around two women for every thousand who are screened regularly.' Leaflets – including *Breast Screening: a Pocket Guide* and *Breast Screening: the Facts* – are produced by the Programme to ensure that women know what screening can and cannot achieve, and to introduce them to the website if they wish for further information.

Thornton[19] has discussed the impact of expert disagreement on harms and benefits on those being invited for screening, and draws attention to the inflated popular notions both of breast cancer risk and of screening effectiveness. She points out that:

> many women with non-invasive and indolent cancers might have gone to their graves in blissful ignorance had it not been for the zealous pursuit of early cancers in a programme that failed to respect the need for honesty and neutrality when presenting the facts.[19]

In a study designed to assess the written information needs of women recalled for further investigation, Austoker and Ong concluded that the amount of information women required was consistently underestimated, and that reassurance was vital in what was inevitably a stressful and distressing situation.[20] The reassuring aspects of information that should be provided are summarised in Table 6.3.

Thornton and colleagues[21] point out that the question of whether the benefits of screening outweigh the harms is essentially a value judgement and that, despite the continuing scientific controversy, decisions about whether or not to participate should be made by women themselves on the basis of full and *understandable* information. They cite one scientific report of a 44% reduction in mortality in women aged 40–69 years,[11] which was headlined in *The Independent* as 'Screening halves breast cancer death rate.' There was no mention in the ensuing article that mortality also fell in those who were not screened, which was attributed to improvements in treatment. These researchers insist that women must be able to understand the potential harms as well as the benefits of the procedure so that they can make an informed choice for which they are prepared to take responsibility. Statistics must be de-mystified and data presented in terms that are easy to understand but not patronising.[22]

In the 15 years since our previous book on screening was published, the risks of breast cancer screening have come more sharply into focus, with the simplistic notion of screening as automatic benefit being robustly challenged. The controversy between sceptics and zealots continues and, without further respectable research evidence, positions are unlikely to change. No one has so far analysed adequately whether resources used for screening could have been better employed in improving treatment.

Table 6.3 Reassuring aspects of information on recall after mammography

---

Receiving a leaflet describing further assessment as well as the recall letter

Being told that 'being recalled is part of routine (or second-stage) screening and that the great majority are found to have normal breasts'

Being told in the recall letter that more information can be obtained by phoning the centre

Being told that the woman could contact the breast care nurse at the centre

Being told when the results can be expected

Source: Austoker and Ong.[20] Reproduced by kind permission of the authors and the publisher.

The fact remains that the national programme is now well established and the political implications of withdrawing it, at least in the short term, make this a most unlikely option. Furthermore, at least some of the reduction in mortality from this disease in recent years is likely to have resulted from the early detection of treatable tumours, even if it is not possible to quantify this precisely.

The National Screening Committee is keeping the programme under scrutiny. The emphasis for the moment, therefore, should surely be on providing accurate, balanced and understandable information to women who are invited to participate, on quality assurance and training of staff involved in the process, and on making the service more accessible and acceptable to specific high-risk groups, such as the socially deprived and ethnic minorities.

Cervical cancer

During the early 1960s, individual district health authorities began to introduce screening for cervical cancer using the Papanicolaou (Pap) smear test. In 1967, the NHS announced a national programme to screen all women over 35 years of age at five-year intervals. The programme has therefore been running for almost 40 years. There have been many problems over this period with regard to the organisation, accountability and commitment of the programme and the variability of provision and quality across the country, and these have been well rehearsed.[23–25]

The programme was re-launched in 1998, and since then much attention has been paid to improving the system. Current policy in the UK is to offer screening to women aged 25–64 years in England and Wales and aged 21–60 years in Scotland at intervals as shown in Table 6.4.

Coverage is difficult to analyse in the same way as for breast cancer, partly because data are not available for the first 10 years, but also because in some years only the number of tests was recorded. Crude analysis suggests that coverage in England is around 80% and has varied only slightly over time. The variation between regions is also slightly smaller than for breast cancer, but with the same regions having lower and higher uptake. In Wales, the coverage has varied between 81% and 86% over the period 1994–2002. In Scotland, over 87% of eligible women have been screened in the past five years, the programme appears to be working well and strict quality standards have been introduced.[26]

As Waggoner[27] has pointed out, cervical cancer is a serious health problem, with almost 500 000 women developing the disease each year worldwide. Most

Table 6.4 Current NSC cervical screening schedules

Age (years)	Screening interval
25	First screening invitation
25–49	Three-yearly screening invitations
50–64	Five-yearly screening invitations
≥ 65	Only those not screened since age 50 years or those with recent abnormal results invited

cases occur in less developed countries where no effective screening systems are available and where treatment options are minimal. In the developed world, by contrast, women with cervical cancer have benefited from early diagnosis and improved treatment of the disease.

Adab and colleagues[28] conducted a study to assess the effectiveness and efficiency of an opportunistic cervical screening system compared with an organised screening programme. The opportunistic system did not perform well, with poor coverage and over-screening of a minority of women contributing to its inefficiency. At best, its effectiveness was found to be equivalent to that of an organised programme with 10-yearly screening and 50% coverage, but at much greater cost.

However, there are a number of questions that need to be addressed.

It is certainly the case that, since the mid-1980s, the incidence of and mortality from cervical cancer in women born since the 1930s in the UK has fallen, and that screening is the most likely explanation for this.

Peto and colleagues[29] have recently suggested that cervical screening has prevented an epidemic that would have killed about one in 65 of all British women born since 1950, and would have culminated in about 6000 deaths per year in the UK. They admit that these are estimates and are subject to 'substantial uncertainty', particularly with regard to the effects of oral contraceptives and condoms and changes in sexual behaviour.

In a commentary on their paper, Etzioni and Thomas[30] advise caution in interpreting this mathematical modelling approach, which needs to be confirmed by a more thorough analysis. It is also undoubtedly true that for each death that has been prevented, very many women have been screened and many have been treated unnecessarily.

The paper by Peto and colleagues provoked considerable reaction in the correspondence column of the *Lancet*.[31] Raffle and Quinn, for example, acknowledge that cervical screening is now remarkably successful. However, they also point out that in the past 'when there was haphazard screening without policy and standards and cervical cancer was a rare disease, it did a considerable amount of harm, as well as some good, at very high cost per cervical death avoided.' They suggest that the same mistake is currently being repeated with prostate cancer.

In contrast to this mathematical modelling approach, the work of Raffle and colleagues is based on actual data from patients in a service setting.[32] In 2003, they reported a study to determine the frequency of different outcomes in women participating in cervical screening. In the context of the screening programme in Bristol, they carried out an analysis of screening records from 348 419 women and modelling of cases of cervical cancer and deaths with and without screening. They summarised their findings as follows.

- In the NHS Cervical Screening Programme, around 1000 women need to be screened for 35 years in order to prevent one death.
- Over 80% of women with high-grade cervical intra-epithelial neoplasia will not develop invasive cancer, but all of them need to be treated.
- For each death that is prevented, over 150 women have an abnormal result, over 80 women are referred for investigation and over 50 women receive treatment.

The main implications of these findings are threefold. First, there is the scale of the problem of over-detection and the need to change the perception of what an abnormal screening result means in order to avoid needless anxiety about borderline changes. Secondly, because of the resources involved and the possibility of harm rather than benefit, it is imperative that the introduction of further cancer screening programmes is based on impeccable evidence. Thirdly, more research attention needs to be focused on the natural history of cervical cancer. Abnormalities that will not progress to invasive cancer should be identified in order to avoid unnecessary removal of organs and the suggestion of potentially harmful chemotherapy and radiotherapy treatments to women who do not need them.

There is currently discussion about the most effective type of screening test. Following pilot studies, the UK national programme is converting to liquid-based cytology (LBC), a new method of preparing cervical samples for cytological examination, over the next five years. The NSC has also been piloting the use of a test for the human papilloma virus (HPV) by LBC with triage of borderline and mildly dyskaryotic cytology specimens at three sites in England.

In a multi-centre study to investigate HPV in addition to routine testing (the HART study), Cuzick and colleagues[33] found that HPV testing was 20% more sensitive than cytology and had a specificity of 95%. They suggest that it might be more cost-effective to use HPV testing as the primary screening test, reserving cytology for those who test positive.

In a commentary on the HART trial, Franco[34] suggests that it can be viewed as a launch pad for future randomised trials to assess the duration of protection conferred by a negative HPV result and the efficacy of a Pap-centred triage approach to those who test positive.

Maissi and colleagues[35] looked at the psychological impact on women of being tested for HPV when smear test results are borderline or mildly dyskaryotic. They found that HPV-positive results were associated with anxiety, distress and concern beyond that associated with the abnormal smear result. Lack of understanding of the meaning of the results was also associated with very high levels of anxiety.

In a systematic review of LBC, Payne and colleagues[36] concluded that this technique could reduce the number of false-negative results (a major limitation of the Pap smear), reduce the number of unsatisfactory specimens and possibly decrease the time required for cytological examination.

However, in a recent French cross-sectional study, Coste and colleagues[37] compared the sensitivity, specificity and inter-observer reliability of conventional cervical smear tests, monolayer or liquid-based cytology and HPV testing in 2585 women. They found that conventional cervical smear testing was superior in terms of low- and high-grade lesions and in populations with a low or high incidence of abnormalities, and they advised that it should not be replaced by the more expensive tests.

Publication of this paper provoked considerable correspondence in the *British Medical Journal*, but the authors defended their findings convincingly in the following terms:

> Our study shows that sampling can be good with conventional smears when gynaecologists are well trained and cooperate with cytology laboratories. This way of improving sampling quality seems to be more cost-effective than replacing conventional smears by monolayers, a

high-tech but costly and ineffective technique, driven by strong commercial pressure from companies and multiform conflicts of interest.[38]

The level of continuing discussion about cervical screening does suggest that it may be time to rethink policy. The frequency of cervical screening remains a controversial question fuelled by the NSC decision to discontinue screening between the ages of 20 and 24 years, and to recommend three-yearly screening for younger women.

In Australia, where a programme was introduced in 1991 to offer Pap smears every two years to women aged 18–70 years who have ever been sexually active, Dickinson[39] suggests that a change is overdue. He recommends a three-year interval with a starting age of 25 years, and questions whether it is ethical to recommend more frequent smears without giving full information and obtaining proper consent.

Wilson and Lester[40] suggest that there is now sufficient evidence to indicate that too many women are being screened too frequently. The resource savings achieved by increasing the screening interval to five years and screening women aged 25–50 years might be better spent on improving the quality of the programme and reaching those women, often the most deprived and marginalised, who have never been screened.

Raffle[41] also questions the decision to continue to offer screening to women over 50 years of age and to shorten the screening interval from five to three years in younger women: 'National decisions on single issues disregard competing needs and force local decision makers to neglect other more pressing problems.' Putting it into perspective, she states:

> you can prevent one death every 22 years by routine five-yearly screening beyond age 50, one death a year and harm an extra 1000 by switching to three-yearly screening under 50, or 10 deaths a year through support that helps smokers stop, and have enough spare to provide first-rate nursing care and family support at home for 183 patients facing death from cancer.[41]

As with breast cancer, the question of improving written information for women about cervical screening is paramount. As Davey and colleagues point out,[42] cervical screening can be a substantial emotional event for women, as well as a rather unpleasant procedure. They conducted a systematic review of the literature to develop evidence-based criteria for the content of letters and leaflets for each stage of the screening process – from invitation for the initial smear test to treatment when required. Several factors, including appropriate content, readability and presentation, are involved in providing high-quality information, and written information should be backed up by access to a healthcare professional, particularly in the case of abnormal or suspicious results.

Better communication of risk can also improve informed uptake of screening. Women overestimate both population and individual risk of cancer, due in no small part to the media interest in and coverage of the topic. Holloway and colleagues[43] conducted a cluster-randomised trial using a risk communication package delivered by nurses in primary care compared with normal screening practice. Those who received a 10-minute counselling session integrated with the smear test appointment were less likely to prefer a shorter screening interval and showed a better knowledge and less anxiety. The extra cost per woman was only £6.

The National Screening Committee is due to review the cervical screening programme when the results of the pilot studies of alternative types of test have been assessed.

It is always going to be both politically and professionally difficult to stop or make radical changes to an established screening procedure, but it does seem to us that there is potential for still better information for the target population, further research on the sensitivity and specificity of the various tests, and a reconsideration both of the age range of those eligible for screening and of screening frequency. There is also the future prospect of automatic machine testing for smears.

In addition, we must acknowledge that in any system as large as the national cervical cancer screening programme – or indeed the breast screening programme – errors are bound to occur. Certain errors are inexcusable – for example, non-reporting of abnormal test results, or excessive delay in reporting results. However, other mistakes, such as misinterpretation of borderline findings, are inevitable. They can be minimised by effective quality control, but it would be unrealistic to expect them to be eradicated.

As Laurence[44] has pointed out in relation to screening for both breast and cervical cancer, 'Medicine is not an exact science. All patients seek certainty but, regrettably, it is only probabilities that are on offer. Screening may reduce the risk of dying of cancer, but it can't eliminate it.'

Colorectal cancer

The second edition of the *American Guide to Clinical Preventive Services* recommended screening for colorectal cancer for everyone aged over 50 years with annual faecal occult blood testing or sigmoidoscopy, or both.[45] At the time of publication, there was insufficient evidence to determine which method was best, or whether a combination of both was more effective.

In 2002, the American Cancer Society produced guidelines for the early detection of cancer, and their recommendations with regard to colorectal cancer are reproduced in Table 6.5.[46]

The European Commission published its *Proposal for a Council Recommendation on Cancer Screening* in 2003.[47,48] For colorectal cancer, it contends that sufficient evidence exists on cost-effectiveness and negative effects to recommend screening at a population level, and that faecal occult blood testing should be offered to men and women aged 50–74 years.

Australia is currently undertaking pilot studies to evaluate the efficacy of a national colorectal screening programme, but firm recommendations are not expected before 2007.[49]

In the UK, the National Screening Committee began a pilot screening programme in 2000, and the results indicated that early detection by screening can reduce mortality from the disease. A working group has been set up to plan the introduction of colorectal cancer screening, and a planning group is currently

Table 6.5 American Cancer Society recommendations for colorectal cancer screening

Cancer site	Population	Test or procedure	Frequency
Colorectal	Men and women aged ≥ 50 years	Faecal occult blood test (FOBT) and flexible sigmoidoscopy or	Annual FOBT and flexible sigmoidoscopy every 5 years starting at age 50 years
		Flexible sigmoidoscopy or	Every 5 years, starting at age 50 years
		FOBT or	Annually, starting at age 50 years
		Colonoscopy or	Every 10 years, starting at age 50 years
		Double-contrast barium enema (DCBE)	Every 5 years, starting at age 50 years

identifying the resources needed for a national programme. Option appraisal of different screening policies has been commissioned from Sheffield University.

Although screening for faecal occult blood has been shown to be efficacious in the context of studies conducted by highly motivated research teams, results in routine clinical practice may not achieve such high levels of performance. For this reason, a demonstration pilot was conducted – on the advice of the NSC – to test the feasibility of a national screening programme for colorectal cancer, and the results of the first round of the project have now been reported.[50,51]

The study was conducted in two areas, namely Coventry and Warwickshire (two English health authorities) and Grampian, Tayside and Fife (three Scottish NHS Boards). Guaiac-based faecal occult blood tests were performed over a two-year period in order to assess whether a national programme would reduce mortality.

The results suggest that the outcomes necessary to obtain a reduction could be achieved by screening in the NHS outside the context of a randomised trial and would be cost-effective. Health ministers in England and Scotland have indicated that national programmes will be introduced, but screening modalities and timescales have yet to be agreed.[52,53]

Other issues, such as uptake, training for screening personnel, and sensitivity and specificity of available tests, still require further consideration, as do frequency of screening, age range of those to be invited and the type of test.[54,55]

While acknowledging the feasibility of the programme, the pilot study group concludes that 'there is little doubt that a screening programme would put further pressure on an already overstretched endoscopy service, and the introduction of screening must go hand in hand with improvements in the provision of services.'[51]

Although bowel cancer is the second commonest cause of death from cancer in the UK and 80% of cases can be successfully treated if detected early, this measured approach is to be applauded, and shows that important lessons have been learned from the difficulties encountered in both the breast and cervical cancer screening programmes.

The NSC will wait for the results of the Sheffield option appraisal study and then review the position before making recommendations on exactly when and how the colorectal screening programme should be implemented. In recent years treatment for colorectal cancer has improved substantially, and new treatments are likely to be available for patients with early as well as advanced disease in the near future.[56] This is a screening programme that, if carefully introduced and properly managed, should make sense.

Prostate cancer

Screening for prostate cancer is the subject of continuing controversy. The incidence of the disease is rising worldwide both because of the growth in the elderly population and because more cases are being diagnosed. Around 20 000 cases of the disease are diagnosed every year (with about 9000 deaths), and 90% of those identified are men aged 65 years or over. The main diagnostic test is the prostate-specific antigen (PSA) test, and digital rectal examination and transrectal ultrasound (TRUS) can also be used, with confirmation by biopsy.

Having reviewed 432 key studies, Selley and colleagues[57] found that many of the criteria for assessing the need for a population programme have not been met for prostate cancer. There is a lack of knowledge about the epidemiology and natural history of the disease, a poor level of accuracy in the screening tests, and a lack of good-quality evidence concerning the effectiveness and cost-effectiveness of treatments for localised prostate cancer.

Selley and colleagues make the following five suggestions for ongoing research.

1 A large-scale randomised controlled trial (RCT) is required to compare radical prostatectomy with conservative management (looking at short- and medium-term outcomes as well as mortality and progression).
2 A full cost-effectiveness analysis is required (i.e. RCT using UK cost data).
3 Further research is required to determine which are the best diagnostic procedures and methods for staging.
4 More information is needed about the natural history of prostate cancer, as well as its aetiology and risk factors.
5 Only when good-quality data become available about the natural history of the disease, optimum screening tests and radical treatments should a full evaluation of the cost-effectiveness of screening be undertaken.

They conclude that current evidence does not support a national screening programme for prostate cancer in the UK, and that there is no justification for the routine use of PSA testing in primary care.

The UK National Screening Committee does not recommend population screening but recognises that, with increased public awareness of the problem, many men may seek the PSA test in the hope of early treatment if the result is positive and reassurance if it is negative. A service to allow people to assess the benefits and harms of the PSA test – the Prostate Cancer Risk Management Programme[58] – has therefore been introduced to provide full information to enable an informed choice, to arrange a PSA test for those who wish for it, and to ensure adequate follow-up as needed.

Donovan and colleagues[59] point out the ambiguity in official advice which states that 'any man considering a PSA test will be given detailed information to enable him to make an informed choice about whether to proceed with a test or not.' They contend that this implies that asymptomatic men may have the test if they wish, so there is ambiguity about whether screening is supported and confusion about what this policy actually means. They fear that prostate cancer screening may creep in by the back door although it does not fulfil the basic criteria for screening, and they suggest that the uncertainties should be very clearly explained, particularly that early detection and treatment of localised prostate cancer is of unproven benefit and may be harmful.

In the second edition of the *American Guide to Clinical Preventive Services*, produced by the US Preventive Services Task Force,[45] routine screening for prostate cancer with digital rectal examination, serum tumour markers (e.g. PSA) or transrectal ultrasound was not recommended. In a 2002 update that recommendation was upheld in the following terms:

> The USPSTF found good evidence that PSA screening can detect early-stage prostate cancer, but mixed and inconclusive evidence that early detection improves health outcomes. Screening is associated with important harms, including frequent false-positive results and unnecessary anxiety, biopsies, and potential complications of treatment of some cancers that may never have affected a patient's health. The USPSTF concludes that evidence is insufficient to determine whether the benefits outweigh the harms for a screened population.[60]

The American Cancer Society, on the other hand, recommends that the PSA test and digital rectal examination should be offered annually from the age of 50 years to men who have a life expectancy of more than 10 years.[46] However, they do also suggest that information should be provided on the benefits and limitations of the test so that men can make an informed decision with the clinician's assistance.

The debate continues and arouses fierce feelings. In 2001, Yamey and Wilkes, then editors of the *Western Medical Journal*, argued in the *San Francisco Chronicle* that there was no good evidence for screening healthy men for prostate cancer. There was a furious backlash, and by the end of the day on which the article appeared their email inboxes were jammed with accusations, abuse and threats.[61] They concluded that 'with the widespread belief in America that every man should know his PSA, a belief driven by politics and not evidence, we fear that sceptical voices like ours will always be drowned out.'

In 2003 in Australia, Professor Alan Coates, chief executive of the Cancer Council Australia, stated that he would not choose to have a PSA test: 'the test may find things that didn't need to be found or it may find things when it is too late to fix them.'[62] This also unleashed a torrent of abuse and accusation from the advocates of screening.

However, the pro-screening approach is not confined to America or Australia. McCartney,[63] a general practitioner in Glasgow, writes of a letter that she received from the Prostate Research Campaign UK, as part of their *Ignorance Isn't Bliss* campaign, asking for her support in displaying posters and leaflets in her surgery encouraging women to use the 'carrot and stick' approach 'to persuade your man to talk to his doctor about his prostate health.' However, as she points out, ignorance about the implications of false positives and false negatives and about unnecessary and invasive tests and treatment is not bliss either. PSA testing remains contentious, and 'no competent adult should be cajoled or manipulated into doing what someone else thinks is best for them – what is required is good, honest information to equip them to make their own decision about risk.'[63]

Commenting on the growth of PSA testing, particularly in the USA, Tannock observes that 'a large number of men who, 15 years ago, would have remained happily unaware of any problem, now have impaired quality of life because they are anxious about their PSA. Such is progress.'[64]

In an American cohort study in two areas of the country, one with much more intensive prostate cancer screening and treatment than the other, no difference in mortality was found over 11 years of follow-up.[65] However, although current evidence argues strongly against routine screening, there is considerable pressure from men's health groups and others for the introduction of screening. One laymen's group in the USA – Us Too! International – which campaigns for PSA screening and has branches in nine countries (including the UK), derives 95% of its funding from the pharmaceutical industry.[66] What such advocates of screening fail to acknowledge, it seems, are the dangers of over-diagnosis of cancers (which, if undetected, would have caused no harm) and over-treatment (with substantial unpleasant consequences such as impotence or incontinence).

In a qualitative study to explore the attitudes of men with confirmed or suspected prostate cancer, Chapple and colleagues found that most such men (48 out of 52 interviewed) strongly advocate PSA testing.[67] The four men who opposed screening had sought information alerting them to the uncertainty about the benefits of treatment, and two regretted being screened. One of these was a 74-year-old man who had had a raised PSA reading and had decided against treatment in favour of watchful waiting: 'I had read up on things and I was terrified of either incontinence or lack of sex. Basically I wish I hadn't known. I would happily have lived on in ignorance.' The authors state that policy makers, politicians and doctors need to understand why people want access to PSA testing so that they can find better ways of communicating risk information.

In commenting on these two studies, Thornton and Dixon-Woods[68] remind us of the ethical dimension of screening and suggest that engaging with the public rather than insisting on the 'rightness' of the science would be a more productive way to reconcile the differences between risk-conscious citizens pressing for screening and authorities being more cautious about its provision.

In a comprehensive review of screening for prostate cancer, Frankel and colleagues conclude that at present there is no scientific case for routine screening outside of research programmes.[69] When it becomes possible to identify high-risk populations and target those men whose cancers are likely to threaten their well-being this situation will change.

The pros and cons of screening for prostate cancer continue to be hotly debated but in our view, with the present state of knowledge, the introduction of a national programme would not be ethical. This is an example of commercial interests being involved in advocating a policy for which there is as yet no evidence, and using their resources for advertising and promotion to increase demand rather than for funding a good-quality research study. There are also cultural, political and media issues involved here.

Other cancers

With the present state of knowledge, there are no other forms of cancer that are currently in serious contention for a national screening programme.

Lung cancer is the most common cause of mortality from cancer in the UK, and is responsible for more than 30 000 deaths a year. Smoking is the main cause of these malignancies, and the incidence of the disease rises rapidly between the ages of 40 and 80 years. Since symptoms do not normally appear until it is too late for curative treatment, it might be supposed that early detection by screening would be helpful. However, the NSC does not recommend screening at present, and the topic will be reviewed in 2006 when the results of major American trials can be considered.

Dalrymple-Hay and Drury, in an overview of screening for lung cancer,[70] cite several trials in the 1970s which showed no improvement in mortality following screening, although these negative results have been attributed to flaws in the design, conduct and analysis of the studies. These studies do not provide sufficient evidence against screening in principle, and the search for a suitable screening tool continues. The three tests that are most likely to fulfil the criteria are chest X-ray, sputum cytology and computed tomography, of which the last is still the subject of research but would seem to hold the most promise.

The Early Lung Cancer Action Project (ELCAP) study in New York – promoted in 2000 by Mayor Rudolf Giuliani to 'help develop the best means for early detection and successful treatment of lung cancer' – is looking at the efficacy of CT screening in early detection. It is studying 10 000 smokers aged 60 years or over with no history of cancer who undergo screening with spiral CT.[71] This method is much more sensitive than chest X-ray or sputum cytology and detects smaller lesions, but there is no control group and thus the findings will not show if the method has any benefits or whether it simply leads to over-diagnosis.

However, Woloshin and colleagues[72] warn that it would be premature and possibly dangerous to move forward with spiral CT screening before a randomised controlled trial has confirmed its safety. There is the real risk of over-diagnosis and unnecessary and invasive follow-up procedures and treatment, and there is no evidence that screening saves lives.

Various studies have failed to show conclusive evidence that screening by any of the current methods reduces mortality from lung cancer, or that the benefits of early detection outweigh the inherent risk of CT. Although spinal CT can detect small pulmonary lesions, 95% of these are benign.[73-76]

Lung cancer is without question a major public health concern, but there are still too many unanswered questions for a routine screening programme to be considered for the present. The US Lung Screening Study (LSS) is currently under way and will randomise high-risk patients to screening CT or conventional chest X-ray.[77]

It is likely, however, that with renewed interest in the subject, particularly in America, public demand for screening will grow. It should be resisted until there is more solid scientific evidence of benefit. The MRC and European groups have put forward proposals for a major randomised controlled study of CT screening which has yet to receive funding.

Ovarian cancer is the seventh commonest cause of cancer in women. For women whose disease at diagnosis is confined to the ovaries, survival is about

75% at 5 years. This has led to interest in the possibility of screening that might result in earlier diagnosis and a reduction in both morbidity and mortality. Current screening methods include ultrasound scanning and the measurement of the tumour marker cancer antigen 125 (CA 125) in serum.

Bell and colleagues conducted a systematic review of screening for ovarian cancer to evaluate the performance of current screening tests, to assess possible adverse effects, to report on the development of newer screening methods and to look at cost-effectiveness in different risk groups.[78] They concluded that further evidence is required before a decision can be made about the potential benefits, harms and costs of a screening programme for this disease.

Three randomised controlled trials are currently ongoing, and the results of the Medical Research Council trial in the UK are awaited before any decisions are taken here. The National Screening Committee's position is that no screening should take place outside this trial, with a review of the position expected by April 2007.

A family history of ovarian cancer is one of the strongest risk factors for the disease, and some UK centres currently offer screening to such women, although there is as yet no agreement about the criteria used to assess risk and no evidence as to whether this policy reduces mortality. Since the consequence of a false-positive result is surgery, it is clearly important to exercise great caution. This is another area where consumer-led demand for screening is likely to increase but should be resisted until firm evidence of benefit is forthcoming.

Skin cancer or melanoma is a significant cause of morbidity and mortality worldwide and its incidence is increasing, with around 46 000 new cases diagnosed each year in the UK.[79]

Helfand and colleagues[80] conducted a comprehensive systematic review of screening for skin cancer for the Agency for Healthcare Research and Quality in the USA in order to examine published data on its effectiveness by a primary care provider. They concluded that the quality of the evidence for routine screening in primary care ranged from poor to fair, but they suggested that screening by means of a risk-assessment technique to identify suspicious pigmented lesions in those at highest risk who were seeing the doctor for another reason might be the most promising strategy for addressing this disease in older adults.

In a cluster randomised controlled trial of population screening for melanoma in Australia, Aitken and colleagues[81] studied a sample of 560 000 adults aged 30 years or over who had been randomly allocated to intervention or control groups. The intervention group received thorough skin self-examination and whole body skin examination by a doctor, with open access to skin-cancer-screening clinics. The control group received normal medical care.

The intervention has been shown to be feasible in practice, with an encouraging level of participation in screening and good cooperation and interest from the communities and doctors involved. However, the authors concede that there is as yet little empirical evidence that a population-based screening programme has the potential to reduce mortality from melanoma. Once again, demand for screening is in danger of increasing in the absence of conclusive scientific evidence of benefit, and without full knowledge of the costs and hazards involved.

Screening for other, less prevalent forms of cancer is not considered appropriate with the present state of knowledge, but the NSC will continue to keep the situation under review. It is organising a workshop on screening for bladder cancer to review occupational screening schemes for those at highest risk. The aim must be to limit cancer-screening services to those types of tumour for which there is unequivocal evidence of benefit, and to resist the pressure from special interest and commercial groups, which will undoubtedly continue and intensify.

Coronary heart disease, stroke and abdominal aortic aneurysm

Cardiovascular and related diseases have taken over from the infectious diseases of the nineteenth century as the main causes of death in the industrialised world. Coronary heart disease (CHD) is the leading single cause of death in the UK.

The National Service Framework for Coronary Heart Disease in England[82] gives priority, for example, to identifying people with CHD for systematic follow-up to offer advice and treatment in order to reduce the risk of recurrence. For those who are not in this high-risk group, the priority is to encourage lifestyle changes such as stopping smoking, amending diet and increasing exercise.

Since diabetes and cardiovascular disease are closely associated, the National Screening Committee has integrated these recommendations with those of the National Service Framework for Diabetes to create the Diabetic, Heart Disease and Stroke Prevention Project, currently being piloted in nine inner-city primary care trusts in England.[83] The results of the pilot will be reviewed during 2006, when national roll-out will be considered.

In 2001, the Scottish Executive established a multi-agency community-based demonstration project in Paisley, a town that has one of the worst heart disease records in the country, but with a long history of community involvement in cardiovascular disease. The Have a Heart Paisley (HAHP) project had four broad aims:[84]

- to change the life and perceptions of every citizen of Paisley by impacting on life circumstances, lifestyle and specific cardiovascular issues
- to prevent heart disease from developing
- to delay the progression of existing heart disease
- to ensure access to appropriate care once symptoms of heart disease are present, and to prevent them from getting worse.

The Scottish Executive stance on the problem of cardiovascular disease in general is that all NHS Boards should, through their Managed Clinical Networks, develop explicit coronary heart disease and stroke prevention strategies. They are expected to adopt a population approach to improving the health of their communities, complemented by a 'high-risk groups approach' targeted at certain groups, such as those with raised blood pressure or cholesterol levels or diabetes, as well as the most socially disadvantaged.

Standard 4 of the National Service Framework for Coronary Heart Disease concerns population cardiovascular risk screening in primary care. However, although CHD is an important preventable health problem in the UK, and reduction of risk factors such as smoking and raised levels of blood pressure and cholesterol has been shown to be effective, Rouse and Adab[85] contend that the National Service Framework standard does not meet the NSC criteria for establishing a population-screening programme. There are no plans for central organisation and coordination, no agreed quality assurance standards and no uniform system of performance assessment. They argue that the benefits of population cardiovascular screening must be established through properly conducted trials and that, if a programme is to be introduced, adequate resources and management structures must first be identified.

McAlister and colleagues[86] conducted a systematic review of secondary prevention programmes in CHD and found that disease management approaches have a positive impact on care and improve both quality of life and functional status. The optimal mix of components and the cost-effectiveness of this approach remain unclear, and since those studied were known to have CHD, it cannot be regarded as screening.

Marteau and Kinmonth[87] stress the importance of informed choice in cardiovascular risk screening. As they point out, categorising individuals can be associated with the adverse effects of labelling and anxiety, and many people do not want to pay the price of monitoring and drug treatment for an uncertain reduction in personal risk. Screening may benefit populations, but only a few individuals will benefit and some may even be harmed by participation. They call for studies to evaluate the impact of a policy of informed choice on reducing cardiovascular risk in high-risk populations identified by screening.

In an editorial commenting on this paper, Brindle and Fahey[88] point to the difficulties of accurate risk assessment in primary care, where only a very few patient records will contain adequate data on risk factors. That aside, they stress the importance of a dialogue between clinician and high-risk patient about possible interventions, but caution that 'until scientific evaluation catches up with political expediency, the goal of involving patients in making genuinely informed choices about coronary heart disease screening seems a long away off.'

Wilson and colleagues[89] compared methods (National Service Framework criteria, Sheffield tables, age threshold of 50 years, estimated risk assessment using fixed cholesterol values) of identifying individuals at increased risk of coronary disease using data from the Health Survey for England on 6307 people aged between 30 and 74 years with no history of myocardial infarction, stroke or angina. They concluded that measuring the cholesterol level of everyone aged 50 years or over would be a simple and efficient way of identifying those at high risk of coronary disease in the population.

This approach was criticised by Assmann and colleagues[90] as being an oversimplification and omitting patients at borderline risk under the age of 50 years. Wilson and colleagues[91] replied that the study was intended to answer a pragmatic question on risk assessment and would help to target cholesterol measurement within the finite budget of the NHS. Although clinicians may not measure cholesterol levels routinely in younger patients, they are unlikely to ignore other important risk factors such as smoking, obesity and blood pressure.

The general practice workload implications of the National Service Framework for CHD are also a cause for concern. Referring to a survey by Hippisley-Cox and Pringle,[92] Toop and Richards suggest that population-based approaches to promoting primary prevention using similar advertising techniques to the tobacco and food industries could be just as effective, if not more so, in encouraging healthy lifestyles as general population screening.[93]

We would agree with the calculations of McPherson and colleagues in their estimation of the impact of changes in risk factors on the incidence of and mortality from CHD as summarised below.[94]

- If everyone were able to reduce and maintain a serum cholesterol level of less than 6.5 mmol/l, the CHD reduction would be around 11%.
- Changes in physical activity could result in an overall reduction of 10% in CHD risk if people who now have lightly active or sedentary lifestyles changed to a moderate level of activity.
- A reduction in diastolic blood pressure to a level below 76 mmHg across the population would result in a 15% reduction in CHD for men and a 12% reduction for women.
- If all those who currently smoke more than 10 cigarettes a day were to cut down to fewer than 10 a day, there could be a 5% drop in CHD. The risk attributable to all smoking, including recent quitters, is 20% for men and 17% for women. Therefore if everyone quit, CHD would be reduced by those percentages.
- Changes in the prevalence of obesity could be responsible for a 3% change in CHD if the prevalence of body mass index over 30 was reduced to 6% among men and 8% among women.
- A moderately optimistic summation of plausible improvements in these risk factors could predict a change in incidence of CHD of around 30% in 10 years.

As Beaglehole[95] has pointed out, the major risk factors for cardiovascular disease and their causes are well known, and in their absence this is a rare cause of death: 'There is now a strong case for diverting scientists, the bodies that fund them, and the journals that publish their work, away from aetiological research and towards the more challenging task of identifying the best ways of enabling people and populations to lower their risk of cardiovascular disease.' It is also important to treat those identified as being at high risk.

Primary prevention with advice on smoking cessation, diet and exercise, rather than population screening, must be the best way forward to reduce the risk of CHD and stroke. Smoking, raised blood pressure, raised cholesterol levels and overweight are universally accepted risk factors that are remediable, and there is evidence that modifying these factors does reduce the risk. Most adults visit their GP at least once a year (and almost all visit at least once in every five years), and this contact should be used to identify those at risk.

Smokers should be advised to stop smoking, and anti-smoking clinics and the use of nicotine substitutes have been shown to be helpful. Blood pressure should be measured at least once every three to five years in those aged 25 years or over. If it is found to be raised (140/85 mmHg or more), measurements should be repeated and anti-hypertensive treatment should be started if necessary. Those considered to be overweight should be given dietary advice. Cholesterol levels should be measured in individuals with one or more of the above risk factors.

National population screening for these risk factors would not be a productive use of resources. The success of this type of screening depends on adequate systems for measurement, advice or treatment as appropriate, and follow-up in primary care.

Abdominal aortic aneurysm

The jury is still out on screening for abdominal aortic aneurysm. A major randomised controlled trial funded by the MRC reported in 2002[96] and provided evidence to support the cost-effectiveness of ultrasound screening in men aged 65–74 years. Greenhalgh and Powell have recently stated that the MRC study supplies the previously missing data to justify a national screening programme.[97]

In a recent population-based randomised controlled trial of ultrasound screening in men aged 65–83 years in Western Australia, Norman and colleagues found that any benefit was almost entirely in the 65–75 years age group. Screening did not reduce overall mortality, and they concluded that the success of screening depends on choice of target age group and the exclusion of ineligible men.[98]

Although the United States Preventive Services Task Force has not updated its 1996 statement that there is insufficient evidence to argue for or against routine screening, Frame suggests that recent studies have added sufficiently to the evidence of benefit from ultrasound screening and elective treatment for aneurysms larger than 55 mm in diameter to justify screening.[99] He cites a report of a population study in Gloucestershire by Earnshaw and colleagues,[100] which found that screening with a simple ultrasound examination reduced mortality after major surgery in men by 42%.

These authors contend that a population-screening programme for men aged 65 years or over based in primary care could save several thousand lives a year at reasonable cost – the scientific arguments are there, and the decision is now political. However, it must also be remembered that the risk from surgery is high, and renal disease can result in a minority of patients.

In commenting on this study, Greenhalgh[101] states that if the results were reproduced nationally, the cost would be less than £50 million per year and ruptured abdominal aortic aneurysm could become a national rarity. He cites the NSC's programme director, Dr Muir Gray, as saying that 'the cost–benefit analysis in the trial is of very high quality, but abdominal aortic aneurysm screening will be delivered effectively and safely only if sufficient resources are made available at local level.'[101]

Further information about the impact of screening on available resources is being sought by the NSC and, as with colorectal cancer, this measured approach is to be commended.

Type 2 diabetes and diabetic retinopathy

In 2001, Wareham and Griffin[102] concluded that, on the basis of the evidence available at the time, there was no justification for universal screening for diabetes in the UK. They advocated rather the optimisation of care of known diabetics and those seen to be at high risk.

Their paper received considerable reaction in the correspondence columns of the *British Medical Journal*. Predictably, Streets (Chief Executive of Diabetes UK) felt that there should be a screening programme, although more evidence was required on how, who and how often to screen.[103] Berger reported on a study in East Germany which concluded that population screening was not effective.[104]

Walker and colleagues pointed out that universal screening would have important implications for resources in primary care.[105]

In reply, Wareham and Griffin[106] restated Cochrane and Holland's view on the ethical imperative of screening, and reiterated the view that further evidence of the effectiveness of screening in reducing mortality and morbidity from type 2 diabetes should be a major research priority.

Spijkeman and colleagues[107] assessed mortality risk in people classified by the Cambridge Risk Score (CRS), a previously validated simple screening tool for undiagnosed type 2 diabetes using information routinely available in primary care. They concluded that individuals who have a positive risk score are at high risk of mortality whether or not subsequent testing shows them to have diabetes, and they suggest that direct public health interventions may be helpful in this population.

The National Screening Committee does not advocate general population screening for diabetes except as part of a peer-reviewed and ethically approved research project. As already mentioned, it is currently piloting the Diabetic, Heart Disease and Stroke Prevention Project in nine primary care trusts in England, with results due in 2006.

There are about 30 million people aged between 40 and 74 years in the UK, of whom about a million are known to have CHD or other forms of vascular disease and a million are known to have diabetes. The main aim of the NSC's risk reduction strategy is to concentrate efforts on these two million while encouraging the remaining 28 million towards a healthy lifestyle. To reduce the burden of CHD, stroke and diabetes for individuals and populations the recommended policy is therefore to ensure that those with known disease receive a comprehensive risk assessment and risk-reduction therapy to reduce blood pressure and cholesterol levels, and support in stopping smoking. Those with type 2 diabetes should have active management of this condition, as well as support in reducing the risk from other factors involved in vascular disease.

The main focus for service delivery is primary care. This is a pragmatic approach to an enormous health problem, and there is already sound evidence to enable a disease control programme to be planned.

Diabetic eye disease is the most common cause of preventable visual loss in people of working age in the UK, and its incidence will continue to increase if, as predicted, the prevalence of type 2 diabetes in 2010 is twice what it was in 1997.

In 2001, Mead and colleagues[108] criticised the current screening practice for diabetic retinopathy as inadequate and inconsistent in terms of both coverage and quality, and estimated that 260 cases of blindness in people aged over 70 years could be prevented each year with systematic screening by photography or ophthalmology.

There has been considerable discussion about the best screening method for diabetic retinopathy. Freudenstein and Verne[109] quoted the recommendations made by Diabetes UK to the NSC that digital retinal photography was the preferred method. Prasad and colleagues[110] recommended screening by optometrists using slit-lamp biomicroscopy as a more reliable and cost-effective way forward.

Clements[111] points out that digital photography offers several advantages in terms of ease of audit and validation, electronic transmission and patient education and motivation. This view is supported by Prince,[112] a general practitioner, who performs screening for diabetic retinopathy by retinal photography as part of a holistic package of diabetic care. He cites the advantages of patient involvement and an electronic link to a local consultant ophthalmologist for advice on particular cases. The rate of referral to secondary care is low, and the cost per patient screened is £32.

Squirrell and Talbot[113] have set out the advantages and disadvantages of the different methods, as summarised in Table 6.6.

Squirrell and Talbot conclude that no single method satisfies all of the requirements, but currently the preferred method is digital photography. As

Table 6.6 Advantages and disadvantages of different methods of screening for diabetic retinopathy

Method	Advantages	Disadvantages
Retinal photography	Effective technique if mydriatic photography is performed with either 35 mm transparencies or digital systems Retinal image can be used in patient education Hard copy can be put in patient record Amenable to audit	High capital set-up costs Difficulties in reaching all patients who need to be screened Need to provide regular training for graders Potential problem retaining motivated personnel for grading
Optometrist screeners	Effective technique if indirect ophthalmoscope/slit-lamp biomicroscope is used Accessible convenient service Offers holistic package of eye care to the patient	Requires an elaborate quality-control mechanism for the system to be audited
Combined methods	Effective techniques Retinal image can be used in patient education Hard copy can be put in patient record Amenable to audit Accessible convenient service Offers holistic package of eye care to the patient Utilises the well-trained, motivated workforce that optometrists represent	High capital set-up costs Camera systems might have to rotate around practices, potentially limiting accessibility of the service

Source: Squirrell and Talbot.[113] Reproduced by permission of the authors and the publisher.

they point out, in any one region the screening programme that is adopted is likely to be a compromise between the efficacy of the method, the existing infrastructure and local expertise.

In terms of a national screening policy in the UK, Scotland has led the way with its recommendation for national screening for diabetic retinopathy. In 2002, the Health Technology Board for Scotland (now part of NHS Quality Improvement Scotland) recommended the introduction of screening for diabetic retinopathy.[114] In 2003, this was endorsed by the Diabetic Retinopathy Screening Implementation Group, which recommends that all patients with diabetes aged 12 years or over should be screened using digital photography, and that this should be fully operational within Scottish NHS Boards by March 2006. Screening will be offered annually in a range of venues, including mobile vans, hospital clinics and by community optometrists. It is estimated that the cost per patient screened will be less than £22.

However, there are many problems with the implementation of the proposed programme. As is so often the case, the reality does not seem to match the rhetoric.

1   Most diabetics are elderly, often with cataract, leading to technical failure. These failures have been estimated as about 20%, which means that examination by slit lamp is essential.
2   Retention and recruitment of staff is a problem, because of boredom.
3   The actual cost per patient is likely to be considerably higher than the £22 estimated.
4   An effective method of referral for comorbidity discovered on examination is crucial.

In March 2004, the NSC reviewed the evidence on screening for sight-threatening diabetic retinopathy, and recommended the introduction over time of screening of all individuals with diabetes over the age of 12 years.[115]

The target in England is that by 2006 a minimum of 80% of diabetics are to be offered screening for the early detection, and treatment where necessary, of diabetic retinopathy as part of a systematic programme that meets national standards. This should rise to 100% coverage of those at risk by the end of 2006. A Project Advisory Group has been set up to steer the development of the programme and to work closely with equivalent groups in the other UK countries in order to ensure consistency. Lessons can certainly be learned from the Scottish scheme and its difficulties, which are discussed in Chapter 9.

The NSC's strategy of a composite preventive and screening programme for the closely related elements of cardiovascular disease in its various manifestations and diabetes and its consequences is, in our view, likely to be the most pragmatic and productive approach in those at risk of or already diagnosed with these conditions.

Chronic obstructive pulmonary disease

Although chronic obstructive pulmonary disease (COPD) is not at present a candidate for screening, it is likely that there will be developments in this area in view of the effective treatments that are becoming available. The National

Institute for Clinical Excellence has recently published guidelines for the diagnosis and treatment of COPD,[116] and the topic is being kept under review.

Mental illness

This is a complex area in terms of screening, and one for which there are at present no routine screening programmes recommended in the UK. We shall consider screening for depression and then look briefly at screening for personality disorder, with regard to alcohol misuse and domestic violence in particular, which have both been the subject of consideration by the NSC.

Depression

Depression is the third commonest reason for consultation in UK general practice, but it can often go unrecognised or be inadequately treated. A 2002 bulletin on *Effective Health Care* on improving the recognition and management of depression in primary care looked at the available evidence and provided a useful summary.[117] From the review it emerged that the routine administration and feedback of questionnaires, such as the General Health Questionnaire, does not improve patient management or outcome in this condition. Multiple interventions, such as case management by practice nurses, clinician education and greater integration with secondary care services, can improve care and outcome, as does the simple intervention of telephone support.

In 1996, the US Preventive Services Task Force found insufficient evidence to recommend routine screening for depression. In an update on the topic in 2002, they concluded that screening adults for depression can improve outcomes so long as there are systems in place to ensure accurate diagnosis and effective treatment and follow-up.[118]

Hickie and colleagues[119] concluded that the evidence is now in favour of the appropriate use of screening tools for depression in adults in primary care. They found that screening does increase the recognition and diagnosis of depression, but again they stress that this must be allied to a commitment to provide coordinated and prompt follow-up in terms of treatment and care.

Arroll and colleagues[120] conducted a study in New Zealand to determine the diagnostic accuracy of two verbally asked questions in screening for depression. They recruited 15 general practices in Auckland in which 670 consecutive patients who were not taking psychotropic drugs were invited to participate in the study and 476 of these patients took part. They found that two verbal questions would detect most cases of depression in this setting, and they had the advantage of brevity over more complicated questionnaires. The questions were as follows.

1 During the past month have you often been bothered by feeling down, depressed or hopeless?
2 During the past month have you often been bothered by little interest or pleasure in doing things?

If the answer to either question was 'yes', the result of screening was considered to be positive.

In an editorial commenting on this paper,[121] Del Mar and Glasziou state that in diagnostic testing 'more is not necessarily better,' and they welcome the development of simple verbal questions which are feasible within the timescale and resources of a general practice consultation. However, they caution that interpreting the answers to questions that are sensitive but not specific is crucial: 'Hence, a negative on both questions makes depression very unlikely, but a positive, even for both questions, means only that we need to explore more fully the possibility of depression, rather than diagnose it on this basis alone.'[121]

George W Bush's recently announced initiative to 'improve mental health services and support for people of all ages with mental illness' through comprehensive screening has received a largely hostile response.[122] Acknowledging that mental illness, including depression, is like any physical disease may be a positive force in reducing the stigma that still exists. However, this is a hugely complex area and there is again a risk of medicalising normal emotional reactions to traumatic life events such as bereavement, divorce, or difficult home or life circumstances.

A study in Tennessee on the use of antipsychotic drugs in children with attention deficit hyperactivity and conduct disorder found that only a minority of the children for whom they were prescribed were in fact psychotic, there was no real evidence of benefit and there were significant side-effects.[123] Dr Daniel Fisher, one of the commissioners involved in producing the report for the president, has expressed concern that widespread screening could result in greater numbers of children being given 'a label, a diagnosis and a medication,' and that mental health problems will continue to be used as a substitute for addressing the social, cultural and economic needs of children.[124]

The NSC does not currently recommend routine screening for depression, although this decision is due for review in 2006. On balance, we feel that there is an argument for an opportunistic approach to identifying depressive illness in adults in primary care. Some GPs, although by no means all of them, are already adept at doing this. There is also a need for awareness of the possibility of false-positive results, over-diagnosis and erroneous labelling, and for effective treatment, counselling and follow-up facilities to be available for those who need them.

Alcohol misuse

In April 2004, the US Preventive Services Task Force recommended screening and behavioural counselling interventions to reduce alcohol misuse in adults.[125]

The UK National Screening Committee, on the other hand, found no evidence to support systematic screening for alcohol problems. If there is clinical suspicion of excessive intake in particular individuals it may be appropriate to investigate, but this is part of good clinical practice rather than screening. The position will be reviewed in 2006.[126]

Domestic violence

In a recent review of screening for family and intimate partner violence, the US Preventive Services Task Force found insufficient evidence to argue for or against screening of parents or guardians for the physical abuse of children, screening of women for intimate partner violence, or screening of older adults, or their carers, for elder abuse.[127]

On the basis of a report commissioned from the Department of Primary Care at the Royal London and Bart's Medical School in 2001, the NSC recommended that screening for domestic violence should not be introduced in the UK. This decision will be reviewed in 2005, and further consideration of the topic is under way within the Children's National Service Framework.

In 2002, Ramsay and colleagues published a systematic review on the subject.[128] They concluded that although domestic violence is a common problem with major health consequences, particularly for women, screening cannot be justified in the absence of evidence for the benefit of specific interventions and the absence of harm.

Goodyear-Smith and Arroll[129] concluded that screening for domestic violence cannot be justified until there is an effective and acceptable test, GPs have training in the skills needed to care for patients in such a situation, and there are appropriate referral programmes for effective management. They suggest that GPs and Accident and Emergency doctors should be aware of the problem and consider this possibility in patients presenting with physical injuries, psychological disturbance or social dysfunction.

Ferris[130] confirms that intimate partner violence is a major public health and human rights issue of which women are overwhelmingly the victims, and that it has enormous implications for wider family well-being. There is an urgent need for further research in the form of trials of the effectiveness of various interventions and for demonstration projects. Until the position becomes clearer, the best approach must be for general practitioners to recognise and respond to the problem by referring those involved to existing facilities such as women's refuges and victim support groups.

The NSC have considered screening for domestic violence in pregnancy and concluded that such screening should not be offered routinely at present and that further research on the effectiveness of existing screening tools is necessary.

The whole area of mental illness in its various guises is still in most ways more difficult to approach than physical illness. Deeply ingrained stigma continues to exist, and the tools for screening are few and rudimentary. Once again, the NSC's measured approach offers the best hope that screening will be introduced only if and when incontrovertible evidence of benefit is available. For now, vigilant case finding in primary care with appropriate follow-up continues to be the best way forward.

Occupational health

Occupational screening in countries such as the UK has changed considerably because of the changes in types of working and attitudes to work. There has been a reduction in many heavy industries, such as coal, steel and chemical production, and the construction, financial and office sectors have increased exponentially. There is thus much less concern with the health effects of industrial processes, such as pneumoconiosis in miners, and more emphasis on lifestyles and good working environments and practices. The trade unions are less powerful in protecting workers in the newer industries, where union membership is no longer mandatory.

The Health and Safety Commission (HSC) and the Health and Safety Executive (HSE) now exist to protect against risks to health or safety arising from work activities, as well as to support research and training and to provide information and advice on occupational issues.

The Health and Safety Executive[131] defines screening or surveillance in the occupational setting as 'putting in place systematic, regular and appropriate procedures to detect early signs of work-related ill health among employees exposed to certain health risks, and acting on the results.'

Rose[132] has suggested five main areas of occupational screening, as summarised in Table 6.7.

In the present context we shall combine Rose's third and fourth categories under the general heading of *ongoing surveillance*.

Fitness for work

Pre-employment health checks are not a legal requirement, but many firms do check an individual's health status and medical history. This pre-employment screening can vary from a simple self-completed questionnaire (designed mainly to protect an employer if an undisclosed chronic health problem subsequently affects performance) to a detailed medical examination and various tests to assess fitness for certain strenuous or potentially dangerous jobs.

Worksite screening

Screening to assess fitness during routine work exposure to a hazard remains relevant, although working conditions in this country are now rigorously

Table 6.7 Five main areas of occupational screening

Area	Category	Examples
1	To assess fitness for task (i) Pre-employment (ii) Pre-placement for specific task	Food handlers, crane operators
2	To assess fitness during routine exposure to hazard	Specific chemicals, noise, radiation, vibration
3	To assess general health risks from history or lifestyle	For general health promotion, such as smoking cessation, for insurance purposes, for entry into pension plan
4	To assess capability	Use of drugs/alcohol pre-employment; routine or random testing during employment, or after a specific incident/accident
5	Genetic screening	Still in infancy in occupational setting, but substantial ethical issues are unresolved

controlled and there are strict guidelines for monitoring exposure in the workplace.

The HSE's regulations 10 and 11 provide detailed monitoring and surveillance guidelines for those working with, for example, known or suspected carcinogens, man-made mineral fibres, or rubber or leather dust. For example, Bollinger and colleagues[133] reported that a screening programme for natural rubber latex (NRL) allergy could identify healthcare workers at risk of dermatitis, who could then be supplied with synthetic gloves to enable them to continue working.

In 2001, the HSC's Advisory Committee on Toxic Substances[134] reported on the value of urinary cytology screening for workers who are or have been exposed to bladder carcinogens by working, for example, with certain dyestuffs, or in rubber or chemical manufacture. They concluded that there was no clear medical justification for such screening, but that employers should be free to offer it if they so wished. If offered, it should be continued after exposure or employment ceases in view of the lengthy latency period between exposure and overt disease. The COSHH* regulations require screening over at least annual intervals for those working with three named aromatic amines and two specific dyestuffs.

The situation seems a little confused, and the NSC is to organise a workshop on bladder cancer screening to review occupational screening schemes for those at highest risk. The policy position will be reviewed thereafter.

Work-related musculoskeletal disorders (WRMSD) are a major cause of sickness absence in the UK, with an estimated 9.9 million working days lost per year as a result. Reducing this was one of the priorities in the HSC's Strategic Plan for 2001–04,[135] but there are no effective screening tools to predict individuals liable to back pain or other muscular injuries, and education of workers in safe lifting techniques and how to avoid repetitive strain injury seem likely to be more productive.

Ongoing surveillance

Some firms run in-house health promotion schemes. Some have regular screening examinations for certain categories of staff, such as airline pilots, and there are various drug and alcohol control programmes in operation. Again these cannot properly be regarded as screening, but rather as human resource issues in occupational health, although there are important factors involved, such as confidentiality and individual autonomy, which should not be ignored.

In the past few years, occupational health has grown in importance as employers and employees and their representatives have recognised the contribution that occupational physicians can make to good management in healthy enterprises. In a recent study of the competencies of occupational physicians, Reetoo and colleagues[136] found that there is still poor understanding of the role of occupational physicians and a low level of occupational health support to British industry. They suggest that existing training schemes for occupational physicians should be reviewed and modified where necessary, awareness of the importance and multi-disciplinary nature of occupational health should be increased, and access to occupational health support should be improved, particularly for small- and medium-sized enterprises.

* Control of Substances Hazardous to Health.

Genetic screening

Genetic screening is not yet in general use in the occupational setting, but it is the subject of considerable debate. There are substantial ethical issues that need to be resolved before it is contemplated, as well as liability and insurance factors. There are many who feel that it would be ethically 'wrong' to screen individuals genetically before employment. On the other hand, it could be considered a duty of protection to screen out people with particular susceptibilities who might be damaged by working with specific substances. The debate must continue. Holtzman,[137] for example, has pointed out that although it is now technically feasible to test workers genetically for susceptibility to a particular industrial process, industry would achieve more at less cost by cleaning up the process or environment.

Screening in occupational health is likely to be examined and developed over the coming years. For the present, there are three salient points on which to focus.

First, the relevance of screening tests must be regularly reviewed to ensure that they are necessary and that they are measuring what they are intended to measure. Secondly, treatment and follow-up must be available for any abnormality that is detected, and minor defects should not be allowed to exclude anyone from employment unnecessarily. There is no point in identifying a condition for which there is no treatment or which is irrelevant to the functioning of individuals, but which will label them with potentially harmful consequences, including anxiety. Thirdly, there must be arrangements for competent management of the data obtained and for proper evaluation of any screening tests. This is particularly important when screening takes place outside the normal healthcare framework. The criteria and principles for sound screening practice apply in this context as much as in any other.

Summary and conclusions

Our recommendations for screening in adults are summarised in Table 6.8.

The national programmes for breast and cervical cancer should be continued but kept under review, with an emphasis on quality control and balanced understandable information to enable women to make a truly informed choice without pressure from healthcare professionals with regard to whether or not to participate. Efforts must also be made to improve coverage of those at highest risk.

A national programme of screening for colorectal cancer by faecal occult blood testing in adults aged 50–74 years is planned, but the NSC's measured approach to implementation is welcome. It is essential that adequate diagnostic, treatment and follow-up facilities are in place before such screening is introduced.

Screening for risk factors for coronary heart disease and stroke should be performed in the primary care setting, with advice, treatment and follow-up being given as appropriate.

In the case of abdominal aortic aneurysm, it now seems clear that ultrasound screening in men aged 65 years or over would reduce mortality from this condition, although the benefit in those aged over 75 years has been questioned.

Table 6.8 Our recommendations for screening in adults

Condition	Comment
Breast cancer	National programme should be continued but kept under close review with emphasis on quality control, staff training and good information
Cervical cancer	National programme should be continued with review of alternative types of tests, age range of those eligible and frequency of screening. Good information should be a priority
Colorectal cancer	National screening programme by faecal occult blood testing for adults aged 50–74 years would be of benefit. Await specific recommendations of NSC before implementation
Abdominal aortic aneurysm	Ultrasound screening of men aged 65 years or over seems a reasonable proposition provided that the necessary resources are in place. Await specific recommendations of NSC before implementation
Diabetic retinopathy	National programme of screening for all diabetics aged over 12 years is being planned and implemented. It is essential to be quite clear about how, when and where screening should take place in order to ensure effective implementation
Risk factors for CHD/ stroke Blood pressure Cholesterol Smoking cessation Weight	Surveillance/case-finding approach in general practice

However, as with colorectal cancer, national implementation must await the certainty that adequate facilities and resources are available.

Diabetic retinopathy screening is already under way, and coverage of all diabetics over the age of 12 years is expected to be achieved by the end of 2006. Close attention must be paid to audit and the need to be absolutely clear about how, when and where to screen. Anecdotal evidence from Scotland suggests that the size of the problem may have been underestimated, and that the reality of implementation does not match up to the rhetoric.

As we have already said, screening in adults is an area ripe for exploitation by the private and commercial sectors. It is essential that the National Screening Committee continues to insist on respectable scientific evidence before recommending any further programmes. Skrabanek's contention, quoted at the beginning of this chapter, that 'medicine has no mandate to be meddlesome in the lives of those who do not need it' remains valid.

References

1 Fitzpatrick M (2001) *The Tyranny of Health*. Routledge, London.
2 National electronic Library for Health/National Screening Committee website, March 2004; www.nelh.nhs.uk/screening/vbls/html
3 Baggott R (2000) *Public Health. Policy and politics*. Macmillan Press, Basingstoke.

4 Shapiro S, Venet W, Strax P *et al.* (1982) Ten- to fourteen-year effect of screening on breast cancer mortality. *J Natl Cancer Inst.* **69**: 349–55.

5 Tabar L, Gad A, Holmberg LH *et al.* (1985) Reduction in mortality from breast cancer after mass screening with mammography. *Lancet.* **ii**: 829–32.

6 Tabar L, Fagerberg G, Gunnar D *et al.* (1989) The Swedish Two-County Trial of mammographic screening for breast cancer: recent results and calculation of benefit. *J Epidemiol Commun Health.* **43**: 107–14.

7 Forrest Report (1987) *Breast Cancer Screening. Report to the Health Ministers of England, Wales, Scotland and Northern Ireland by a Working Group chaired by Sir Patrick Forrest.* HMSO, London.

8 Hann A (1996) *The Politics of Breast Cancer Screening.* Ashgate Publishing Co., Aldershot.

9 www.cancerscreening.nhs.uk/breastscreen/statistics.html

10 www.nhshealthquality.org/nhsqis/files/breast_overview.pdf

11 Tabar L, Yen M-F, Vitak B, Chen H-HT, Smith RA and Duffy SW (2003) Mammography service screening and mortality in breast cancer patients: 20-year follow-up before and after introduction of screening. *Lancet.* **361**: 1405–10.

12 Nystrom L, Andersson I, Bjurstam N, Frisell J, Nordenskjold B and Rutqvist LE (2002) Long-term effects of mammography screening: updated overview of the Swedish randomised trials. *Lancet.* **359**: 909–19.

13 Blanks RG, Moss SM, McGahan CE, Quinn MJ and Babb PJ (2000) Effect of NHS breast screening programme on mortality from breast cancer in England and Wales 1990–98: comparison of observed with predicted mortality. *BMJ.* **321**: 665–9.

14 Botha JL, Bray F, Sankila R and Parkin DM (2003) Breast cancer incidence and mortality trends in 16 European countries. *Eur J Cancer.* **39**: 1718–29.

15 Olsen O and Gøtzsche PC (2001) Screening for breast cancer with mammography (Cochrane Review). In: *The Cochrane Library. Issue 4.* Update Software, Oxford.

16 Baum M (2004) Commentary: false premises, false promises and false positives – the case against mammographic screening for breast cancer. *Int J Epidemiol.* **33**: 66–7.

17 Freedman DA, Petitti DB and Robins JM (2004) On the efficacy of screening for breast cancer. *Int J Epidemiol.* **33**: 43–55.

18 *Breast Screening Programme Annual Review 2002*; www.cancerscreening.nhs.uk

19 Thornton H (2003) Mammographic screening: give us the facts. *J R Soc Med.* **96**: 409–10.

20 Austoker J and Ong G (1994) Written information needs of women who are recalled for further investigation of breast screening: results of a multi-centre study. *J Med Screen.* **1**: 238–44.

21 Thornton H, Edwards A and Baum M (2003) Women need better information about routine mammography. *BMJ.* **327**: 101–3.

22 Thornton H, Edwards A and Baum M (2003) Women need better information about routine mammography (letter). *BMJ.* **327**: 869.

23 Roberts A (1982) Cervical cytology in England and Wales 1965–1980. *Health Trends.* **14**: 41–3.

24 Richards T (1985) Poor organisation and lack of will have caused the failure of cervical cancer screening. *BMJ.* **291**: 1135.

25 Holland WW and Stewart S (1990) *Screening in Health Care: benefit or bane?* The Nuffield Provincial Hospitals Trust, London.

26 NHS Quality Improvement Scotland (2003) *Cervical Screening: national overview*; www.nhshealthquality.org

27 Waggoner SE (2003) Cervical cancer. *Lancet.* **361**: 2217–25.

28 Adab P, McGhee SM, Yanova J, Wong CM and Hedley AJ (2004) Effectiveness and efficiency of opportunistic cervical cancer screening: comparison with organised screening. *Med Care.* **42**: 600–9.

29 Peto J, Gilham C, Fletcher O and Matthews FE (2004) The cervical cancer epidemic that screening has prevented in the UK. *Lancet.* **364**: 249–56.

30 Etzioni R and Thomas DB (2004) Modelling the effect of screening for cervical cancer on the population (comment). *Lancet.* **364**: 224–6.

31 Various (2004) Harms and benefits of screening to prevent cervical cancer (correspondence). *Lancet.* **364**: 1483–6.

32 Raffle AE, Alden B, Quinn M, Babb PJ and Brett MT (2003) Outcomes of screening to prevent cancer: analysis of cumulative incidence of cervical abnormality and modelling of cases and deaths prevented. *BMJ.* **326**: 901–4.

33 Cuzick J, Szarewski A *et al.* (2003) Management of women who test positive for high-risk types of human papillomavirus: the Hart Study. *Lancet.* **362**: 1871–6.

34 Franco EL (2003) Are we ready for a paradigm change in cervical cancer screening? *Lancet.* **362**: 1863–4.

35 Maissi E, Marteau TM *et al.* (2004) Psychological effect of human papillomavirus testing in women with borderline or mildly dyskaryotic cervical smear test results: cross-sectional questionnaire study. *BMJ.* **328**: 1293.

36 Payne N, Chilcott J and McGoogan E (2000) Liquid-based cytology in cervical screening: a rapid and systematic review. *Health Technol Assess.* **4**(18); www.hta.nhs web.nhs.uk/execsumm/summ418.htm

37 Coste J, Cochand-Priollet B, de Cremoux P *et al.* (2003) Cross-sectional study of conventional cervical smear, monolayer cytology, and human papillomavirus DNA testing for cervical cancer screening. *BMJ.* **326**: 733.

38 Coste J, Cochand-Priollet B, de Cremoux P *et al.* (2003) Cervical cancer screening. Letter (authors' reply). *BMJ.* **327**: 162.

39 Dickinson JA (2002) Cervical screening: time to change the policy. *Med J Aust.* **176**: 547–50.

40 Wilson S and Lester H (2002) How can we develop a cost-effective quality cervical screening programme? *Br J Gen Pract.* **52**: 485–90.

41 Raffle AE (2004) Cervical screening (editorial). *BMJ.* **328**: 1272–3.

42 Davey C, Austoker J and Jansen C (1998) Improving written information for women about cervical screening: evidence-based criteria for the content of letters and leaflets. *Health Educ J.* **57**: 263–81.

43 Holloway RM, Wilkinson C, Peters TJ *et al.* (2003) Cluster-randomised trial of risk communication to enhance informed uptake of cervical screening. *Br J Gen Pract.* **53**: 620–25.

44 Laurence J (2001) Does screening really save lives? *The Independent.* 7 November.

45 US Preventive Services Task Force (1996) *American Guide to Clinical Preventive Services* (2e). Williams and Wilkins, Baltimore, MD.

46 Smith RA, Cokkinides V, von Eschenbach AC *et al.* (2002) American Cancer Society Guidelines for the Early Detection of Cancer. *CA Cancer J Clin.* **52**: 8–22.

47 Commission of the European Communities (2003) *Proposal for a Council Recommendation on Cancer Screening.* Commission of the European Communities, Brussels.

48 Advisory Committee on Cancer Prevention (2000) Recommendations on cancer screening in the European Union. *Eur J Cancer* **36**: 1473–8.

49 Baker PG (2004) Screening for colorectal cancer – benefit or burden? *J R Coll Physicians Edinb.* **34**: 99–103.

50 www.cancerscreening.nhsuk/colorectal/links.html

51 UK Colorectal Cancer Screening Pilot Group (2004) Results of the first round of a demonstration pilot of screening for colorectal cancer in the United Kingdom. *BMJ.* **329**: 133.

52 www.infodoh.gov.uk/doh/intpress.nsf/page2003–0047

53 Scottish Executive Health Department (2004) *Cancer in Scotland. Action for change. Bowel Cancer Framework for Scotland.* Scottish Executive Health Department, Edinburgh.

54 Schofield JH and Moss S (2003) Screening sigmoidoscopy for colorectal cancer. *Lancet.* **362**: 1167–8.

55 Newcomb PA, Storer BE, Morimoto LM and Templeton A (2003) Long-term efficacy of sigmoidoscopy in reduction of colorectal cancer incidence. *J Natl Cancer Inst.* **95**: 622–5.

56 Slevin M and Payne S (2004) New treatments for colon cancer (editorial). *BMJ.* **329**: 124–6.

57 Selley S, Donovan J, Faulkner A, Coast J and Gillatt D (1997) Diagnosis, management and screening of early localised prostate cancer. *Health Technol Assess.* **1**(2); www.ncchta.org/execsumm/summ102.htm

58 NHS Cancer Screening Programmes (2002) *Prostate Cancer Risk Management Programme: an information pack for primary care.* NHS Cancer Screening Programmes, Sheffield; www.nelc.org.uk

59 Donovan JL, Frankel SJ, Neal DE and Hamdy FC (2001) Screening for prostate cancer in the UK. *BMJ.* **323**: 763–4.

60 www.ahrq.gov/clinic/cps3dix.htm

61 Yamey G and Wilkes M (2002) The PSA storm. *BMJ.* **324**: 431.

62 Chapman S (2003) Fresh row over prostate screening. *BMJ.* **326**: 605.

63 McCartney M (2004) Screening must remain a free choice. *BMJ.* **328**: 1023.

64 Tannock IF (2002) Eradication of a disease: how we cured symptomless prostate cancer (viewpoint). *Lancet.* **359**: 1341–2.

65 Lu-Yao G, Albertsen PC, Stanford JL *et al.* (2002) Natural experiment examining impact of aggressive screening and treatment on prostate cancer mortality in two fixed cohorts from Seattle area and Connecticut. *BMJ.* **325**: 740.

66 Lenzer J (2003) Lay campaigners for prostate screening are funded by industry (news). *BMJ.* **326**: 680.

67 Chapple A, Ziebland S, Shepperd S *et al.* (2002) Why men with prostate cancer want wider access to prostate-specific antigen testing: qualitative study. *BMJ.* **325**: 737–9.

68 Thornton H and Dixon-Woods M (2002) Prostate-specific antigen testing for prostate cancer (editorial). *BMJ.* **325**: 725–6.

69 Frankel SJ, Davey Smith G, Donovan J and Neal D (2003) Screening for prostate cancer. *Lancet.* **361**: 1122–8.

70 Dalrymple-Hay MJR and Drury NE (2001) Screening for lung cancer. *J R Soc Med.* **94**: 2–5.

71 Sone S, Li F, Yang Z *et al.* (2001) Results of three-year mass screening programme for lung cancer using mobile low-dose spiral computed tomography scanner. *Br J Cancer.* **84**: 25–32.

72 Woloshin S, Schwartz LM and Welch HG (2002) Tobacco money up in smoke? Viewpoint. *Lancet.* **359**: 2108–11.

73 Black WC and Welch HG (1997) Screening for disease. *Am J Roentgenol.* **168**: 3–11.

74 Manser RL, Irving LB, Stone C *et al.* (eds) (2001) Screening for lung cancer (Cochrane Review). In: *The Cochrane Library* (4e). Update Software, Oxford.

75 Swensen SJ, Jett JR, Sloan JA *et al.* (2002) Screening for lung cancer with low-dose spiral computed tomography. *Am J Resp Crit Care Med.* **165**: 508–13.

76 Pastorino U, Bellomi M, Landori C *et al.* (2003) Early lung cancer detection with spiral CT and positron emission tomography in heavy smokers: 2-year results. *Lancet.* **362**: 593–7.

77 Heffner JE and Silvestri G (2002) CT screening for lung cancer: is smaller better? *Am J Resp Crit Care Med.* **165**: 433–7.

78 Bell R, Petticrew M, Luengo S and Sheldon TA (1998) Screening for ovarian cancer: a systematic review. *Health Technol Assess.* **2**(2); www.hta.nhsweb.nhs.uk/execsumm/summ202.htm

79 www.cancerresearchuk.org

80 Helfand M, Mahon S and Eden K (2001) *Screening for Skin Cancer.* AHRQ Publication No. 01-S002. Agency for Healthcare Research and Quality, Rockville, MD.

81 Aitken JF, Elwood JM, Lowe JB, Firman DW, Balanda KP and Ring IT (2002) A randomised trial of population screening for melanoma. *J Med Screen.* **9**: 33–7.

82 Department of Health (2000) *National Service Framework for Coronary Heart Disease.* Department of Health, London.

83 www.nelhnhs.uk/screening/adult_pps/dhdreducingrisks.html

84 www.show.scot.nhs.uk/hahpregister/CHDCompare.htm/

85 Rouse A and Adab P (2001) Is population coronary heart disease screening justified? A discussion of the National Service Framework for coronary heart disease (Standard 4). *Br J Gen Pract.* **51**: 834–7.

86 McAlister FA, Lawson FME, Teo KK and Armstrong PW (2001) Randomised trials of secondary prevention programmes in coronary heart disease: systematic review. *BMJ.* **323**: 957–62.

87 Marteau T and Kinmonth L (2002) Screening for cardiovascular disease: public health imperative or matter for individual informed choice? *BMJ.* **325**: 78–80.

88 Brindle P and Fahey T (2002) Primary prevention of coronary heart disease – unevaluated screening inhibits informed choice. *BMJ.* **325**: 56–7.

89 Wilson S, Johnston A, Robson J *et al.* (2003) Comparison of methods to identify individuals at increased risk of coronary heart disease from the general population. *BMJ.* **326**: 1436.

90 Assman G, Cullen P and Schulte H (2003) Methods to identify increased risk of coronary disease in the general population. Conclusion is oversimplification (letter). *BMJ.* **327**: 619.

91 Wilson S *et al.* (2003) Methods to identify increased risk of coronary disease in the general population (authors' reply). *BMJ.* **327**: 619.

92 Hippisley-Cox J and Pringle M (2001) General practice workload implications of the National Service Framework for Coronary Heart Disease: cross-sectional survey. *BMJ.* **323**: 269–70.

93 Toop L and Richards D (2001) Preventing cardiovascular disease in primary care. Targets are fine in principle, but unrealistic (editorial). *BMJ.* **323**: 246–7.

94 McPherson K, Britton A and Causer L (2002) *Coronary Heart Disease: estimating impact of changes in risk factors.* National Heart Forum, London.

95 Beaglehole R (2001) Global cardiovascular disease prevention: time to get serious. *Lancet.* **358**: 661–3.

96 Multicentre Aneurysm Screening Study Group (2002) Multicentre Aneurysm Screening Study (MASS): cost-effectiveness analysis of screening for abdominal aortic aneurysms based on four-year results from randomised controlled trial. *BMJ.* **325**: 1135–8.

97 Greenhalgh RM and Powell JT (2002) Screening men for aortic aneurysm (editorial). *BMJ.* **325**: 1123–4.

98 Norman PE, Jamrozik K, Lawrence-Brown MM *et al.* (2004) Population-based randomised controlled trial on impact of screening on mortality from abdominal aortic aneurysm. *BMJ.* **329**: 1259–62.

99 Frame PS (2004) Screening for abdominal aortic aneurysm. Its time has come (editorial). *BMJ.* **329**: 311–12.

100 Earnshaw JJ, Shaw E, Whyman MR, Poskitt KR and Heather BP (2004) Screening for abdominal aortic aneurysms in men. *BMJ.* **328**: 1122–4.

101 Greenhalgh RM (2004) National screening programme for aortic aneurysm. *BMJ.* **328**: 1087–8.

102 Wareham NJ and Griffin SJ (2001) Should we screen for type 2 diabetes? Evaluation against National Screening Committee criteria. *BMJ.* **322**: 986–8.

103 Streets P (2001) Undiagnosed diabetes must be detected (letter). *BMJ.* **323**: 453.

104 Berger M (2001) Population screening was not effective in former East Germany (letter). *BMJ.* **323**: 453.

105 Walker M, Thomson A and Whincup PH (2001) Screening would have important resource implications for primary care (letter). *BMJ.* **323**: 453.

106 Wareham NJ and Griffin SJ (2001) Authors' reply. *BMJ.* **323**: 453.

107 Spijkeman A, Griffin S, Dekker J, Nijpels G and Wareham NJ (2002) What is the risk of mortality for people who are screen-positive in a diabetes screening programme but who do not have diabetes on biochemical testing? Diabetes screening programmes from a public health perspective. *J Med Screen.* **9**: 187–90.

108 Mead A, Burnett S and Davey C (2001) Diabetic retinal screening in the UK. *J R Soc Med.* **94**: 127–9.

109 Freudenstein U and Verne J (2001) A national screening programme for diabetic retinopathy. Need to learn the lessons of existing screening programmes (editorial). *BMJ.* **323**: 4–5.

110 Prasad S, Swindlehurst H and Clearkin LG (2001) Screening by optometrists is better than screening by fundus photography (letter). *BMJ.* **323**: 998.

111 Clements C (2001) Digital image may be better for screening (letter). *BMJ.* **324**: 849.

112 Prince CB (2001) Screening by retinal photography offers holistic package of diabetic care (letter). *BMJ.* **324**: 849.

113 Squirrell DM and Talbot JF (2003) Screening for diabetic retinopathy. *J R Soc Med.* **96**: 273–6.

114 Facey K, Cummins E, Macpherson K, Morris A, Reay L and Slattery J (2002) *Organisation of Services for Diabetic Retinopathy Screening in Scotland.* Health Technology Report 1. Health Technology Board for Scotland, Glasgow; www.nshhealthquality.org

115 www.nelh.nhs.uk/screening/adult_pps/diabetic_retinopathy.html

116 National Institute for Clinical Excellence (2004) *Chronic Obstructive Pulmonary Disease. Information for people with chronic obstructive pulmonary disease, their families and carers and the public.* National Institute for Clinical Excellence, London.

117 University of York NHS Centre for Reviews and Dissemination (2002) Improving the recognition and management of depression in primary care. *Effect Health Care.* **7**(5): 1–12.

118 www.ahrq.gov/clinic/3rduspstf/depression/depressrr.htm

119 Hickie IB, Davenport TA and Ricci CS (2002) Screening for depression in general practice and related medical settings. *Med J Aust.* **177**: S111–16.

120 Arroll B, Khin N and Kerse N (2003) Screening for depression in primary care with two verbally asked questions: cross-sectional study. *BMJ.* **327**: 1144–6.

121 Del Mar C and Glasziou P (2003) How many conditions can a GP screen for? Editorial. *BMJ.* **327**: 1117.

122 Twisselmann B (2004) Bush plans to screen whole US population for mental illness. Summary of responses. *BMJ.* **329**: 292–3.

123 Cooper WO, Hickson GB, Fuchs C, Arbogast PG and Ray WA (2004) New users of antipsychotic medications among children enrolled in TennCare. *Arch Pediatr Adolesc Med.* **158**: 753–9.

124 Lenzer J (2004) Bush launches controversial mental health plan. News. *BMJ.* **329**: 367.

125 www.ahcpr.gov/clinic/uspstf/uspsdrin.htm

126 www.nelh.nhs.uk/screening/adult_pps/alcohol.html

127 www.ahcpr.gov/clinic/uspstf/uspsfamv.htm

128 Ramsay J, Richardson J, Carter YH, Davidson LL and Feder G (2002) Should health professionals screen women for domestic violence? Systematic review. *BMJ.* **325**: 314

129 Goodyear-Smith and Arroll B (2003) Screening for domestic violence in general practice: a way forward? *Br J Gen Pract.* **53**: 515–18.

130 Ferris LE (2004) Intimate partner violence (editorial). *BMJ.* **328**: 595–6.

131 www.hse.gov.uk/

132 Rose F (2002) Personal communication.

133 Bollinger ME, Mudd K, Keible LA, Hess BL, Bascom R and Hamilton R (2002) A hospital-based screening programme for natural rubber latex allergy. *Ann Allergy Asthma Immunol.* **88**: 560–67.

134 Health and Safety Commission Advisory Committee on Toxic Substances (2001) *Urinary Cytology Screening.* HSC Paper Number ACTS/20/2001. Health and Safety Commission, London.

135 Health and Safety Commission (2001) *HSC Strategic Plan 2001–2004. Priority Programmes*; www.hse.gov.uk/aboutus/plans/hscplans/plan0104–05.htm

136 Reetoo KN, Harrington JM and Macdonald EB (2004) *Competencies of Occupational Physicians*. Report prepared by the University of Glasgow for the Health and Safety Executive and the EEF – the Manufacturers' Organisation. University of Glasgow, Glasgow.

137 Holtzman NA (1996) Medical and ethical issues in genetic screening – an academic view. *Environ Health Perspect.* **104 (Suppl. 5)**: 987–90.

Chapter 7

Screening in the elderly

Old age is the most unexpected of all things that happen.*

Introduction

The 2001 Census[1] showed that for the first time there are more people aged over 60 years in the population of the UK than there are under 16 years, and there has also been an increase in the proportion of people aged over 85 years (*see* Table 7.1).

This ageing of the population reflects longer life expectancy as a result of improvements in standards of living and healthcare. It is also the case that in the last half of the twentieth century there were no major aggressive events, such as the two World Wars, to cause premature mortality during the period.

In 1999, the Royal Commission on Long-Term Care stressed that old age should be seen as an opportunity rather than a problem: 'while physical or mental faculties may change, people should not necessarily be assumed to be passive recipients of the goodwill of others or inevitably incapacitated, befuddled or redundant.'[2] As old age comes to increasing numbers of the population it should be seen as a natural part of life, and not as a burden.

The Commission presented two main arguments in favour of preventive strategies for older people. First, they can delay the onset of disease and disability and thus postpone the need for costly healthcare interventions. Secondly, they can improve the well-being and quality of life of this age group.

They stressed the need for further longitudinal research to 'track the processes and outcomes of preventive interventions and to assess their impact both on quality of life and long-term costs.' However, Clark[3] points out that such research is not encouraged by present funding arrangements and that the selection of outcome measures might vary considerably according to which discipline was leading the work. Many doctors, for example, would focus on the reduction of mortality and the avoidance of a long period of dependence and disability as desired outcomes. Health visitors, on the other hand, would be likely to look at outcomes such as autonomy, independent decision making and improved confidence and self-esteem, which are much more difficult to measure but no less important. Clark poses the following relevant question: 'Has any research sought to identify which outcomes older people themselves would select as indicators of effective services?'[3]

In current census and pension terms at least, old age in the UK officially begins at the age of 60 years for women and 65 years for men, although the Government is considering postponing pensionable age. Clearly many people at these ages are in good or reasonable health and continue to work or to lead productive lives

* Leon Trotsky

Table 7.1 Census data on the UK's ageing population

Proportion of population aged under 16 years	Proportion of population aged 60 years or over	Proportion of population aged 85 years or over
1951		
24%	16%	0.4%
2001		
20%	21%	1.9%

pursuing interests and activities in their increased leisure time. It seems reasonable, therefore, to divide 'old age' into at least three stages, namely *young old age* (60–74 years), *old age* (75–85 years) and *old old age* (over 85 years). Of course this is a very arbitrary division, but offering preventive services to those in the first stage may help them to delay or cope better with many of the inevitable 'rustings' of the ageing process.

It is also the case that although current emphasis is on trying to help people to remain in their own homes or in sheltered housing for as long as possible, those who due to mental and/or physical frailty have to be cared for in a residential home or in hospital have different needs and should not be neglected. In this chapter, however, we shall be concentrating on screening in the community

Is screening of benefit to the elderly?

Views on this issue remain mixed. Because of the relative lack of reputable studies, there is little scientific evidence to support the benefits of screening in this age group, usually because the aims are not clearly stated. There is confusion in the minds of many about the benefits that are sought for the elderly compared with the middle-aged or the young.

Freedman and colleagues,[4] in a study of the immediate effect of a single screen, concluded that there was little treatable and undiagnosed illness in the group studied and that 'the relatively small returns from the very considerable expenditure of effort, time and money convinced us that routine screening of this nature is not justified.'

However, many workers have stressed that identification of disabilities such as hearing loss or reduced mobility can make a considerable difference to older people's enjoyment of life. For example, Tulloch and Moore[5] considered that 'the real pathology of old age is pain, disablement, frustration, boredom, lack of purpose, and loss of identity and self-respect, all of which lead to dissatisfaction with the quality of life.'

In a randomised controlled trial conducted over a period of three years in Denmark, Hendriksen and colleagues[6,7] showed reduced mortality resulting from a programme of home visits at three-monthly intervals that led to an increase in the provision of home helps and equipment and modifications to the home. They estimated the increased cost of visits to be around £600 per person over three years (at 1982 prices), but calculated that savings in terms of the costs of bed days in hospital, months in nursing homes and emergency home services amounted to £1200 per individual.

The work of Khaw and colleagues in the EPIC-Norfolk arm of a European prospective population study in ten countries (EPIC) involves a cohort of 30 000 men and women aged 45–79 years, and seeks to identify potential interventions to maintain health in the ageing population.[8–10] The focus of the study is on identifying major health problems in the ageing population and underlying causes of common and chronic diseases, with a view to designing simple interventions, such as changes in diet and exercise, in order to improve outcomes.

Although screening in this age group will always have its opponents and its advocates, this is in our view a complex and important stage of the life cycle for screening and healthcare, since many of the difficulties encountered (e.g. impairments of sight, hearing, mental health or mobility) can with proper care and surveillance be helped if not cured. A flexible system of surveillance and case finding in primary care would seem to be the most practical way of identifying those individuals who could benefit from further assessment.

Case finding in primary care

The National Service Framework for Older People[11] included a recommendation that elderly people should receive some form of single assessment 'matched to their individual circumstances,' a process which can be carried out either by postal questionnaire or face to face.

Since 1990, primary care teams have been required to offer an annual screening assessment to all patients over the age of 75 years. The terms of the 1990 Contract for General Practice in the National Health Service[12] included the expectation that GPs or other members of the practice team would offer these patients a home visit at least annually to see the home environment. This would include finding out whether carers and relatives are available, social assessment (lifestyle, relationships), mobility assessment (walking, sitting, use of aids), mental assessment, assessment of senses (hearing and vision), assessment of continence, general functional assessment and review of medication.

The new contract for general practitioners[13] which came into force in April 2004 states that these checks will still be available for individuals aged 75 years or over, but only if patients request them. Practices will no longer have to invite patients in this age group for assessment, although many may choose to continue to do so. In practice this flexible approach seems sensible, since many elderly people are independent, have good family or social support and will seek advice or help when they feel that they need it, but it may overlook those who lead lonely, isolated lives.

Table 7.2 Average number of NHS GP consultations per person per year for men and women in three age groups in the year 2000[16]

Age range (years)	Men	Women
45–64	5	5
65–74	6	7
≥ 75	6	7

Table 7.3 Average number of consultations with a practice nurse per person per year for men and women in three age groups in the year 2000[17]

Age range (years)	Men	Women
45–64	1	2
65–74	3	3
≥75	3	3

Recent data on GP consultations for men and women in the relevant age groups are shown in Table 7.2, and it has been suggested that over 90% of those aged over 75 years see their general practitioner at least once a year.[14,15]

The average number of consultations with a practice nurse in the same age groups is shown in Table 7.3.

Thus a system of opportunistic case finding by the primary care team, if implemented effectively (taking advantage of modern information technology which can easily identify those who require surveillance) could reach most people at this stage of the life cycle. The minority of isolated and vulnerable elderly patients who most require assessment but may not ask for it must not be neglected. These individuals are likely to be a small proportion of patients on an average practice list, and could be targeted for assistance from district nurses and/ or social work departments as appropriate.

Buckley and Williamson[18] have suggested that case finding in primary care should be carried out in two stages. The first stage would involve identification of those at high risk who are likely to benefit from the second stage, namely detailed assessment of function.

Freer[19] is among those who have demonstrated the feasibility of opportunistic case finding in the elderly. He contended that the lack of evidence to support formal screening in this age group does not reduce the value of a 'preventive and anticipatory component to primary care' at this time of life. A number of short screening schedules have been developed for use by doctors, nurses, lay people or patients themselves and can help to identify those who would benefit from full assessment. In Freer's pilot study in general practice, only 28 of the 102 patients involved required follow-up, and the system was found to be easy to cope with during normal surgery appointments.

There is still uncertainty about the best way of administering an initial screening questionnaire. For example, Van Haastregt and colleagues[20] found that a programme of home visits aimed at reducing falls and impairments in mobility in elderly people at risk living in the community was not effective, at least in the Dutch healthcare setting.

In a randomised comparison of three methods for administering a screening questionnaire to elderly people, Smeeth and colleagues[21] studied almost 33 000 people aged 75 years or over who were registered with 106 general practices. The methods were postal questionnaire, interview by a layperson (usually a member of the practice clerical staff) and interview by a nurse (usually a practice nurse).

The results showed that postal questionnaires produced a higher response rate than personal interviews but also had higher proportions of missing data. Interviews by nurses, and to a lesser extent interviews by lay interviewers, were associated with lower levels of self-reported morbidity than the postal questionnaires.

The research team suggests that the use of a postal questionnaire is supported by the higher response rate and lower costs of this method. The trial continues and is examining whether the differences observed between the three methods affect the outcomes of mortality, hospital admission rates and quality of life.

However, Clark[3] warns that although randomised controlled trials are the most rigorous method of assessing the effectiveness of medical interventions, they may not be appropriate for evaluating services such as home visiting, which is a complex social interaction rather than a treatment programme. This view has been echoed in a recent study by Thomson and colleagues on evaluating the health effects of social interventions.[22] They state that although randomisation of a social intervention may be possible using natural delays, adding delays for the sole purpose of health research is unethical. They contend that when randomised or other controlled trials are not ethically possible, uncontrolled studies may have to be regarded as good enough, so long as care is taken in the selection of comparison groups.

Conditions to be screened for

There are mixed views on whether to screen for disease or disability, or both, in this age group. Williamson *et al.*[23] suggest that we should screen for loss of physical, mental, social and family function. However, Bulpitt and colleagues[24] state that it may be rather artificial to differentiate between functional disorders and underlying diseases: 'It is preferable to detect hypothyroidism before it leads to dementia, although it is almost certainly still desirable to detect dementia when due to this condition. Functional disorder may be accelerated when the underlying disease process has not been detected or treated.' They advocate screening for both disease and disability, and this seems appropriate in the primary care setting – where a patient is seen as an individual rather than as a set of separate body parts and functions.

Conditions should be considered for screening if they are common and potentially treatable. Many serious physical problems may well have been diagnosed previously, although this is by no means always the case. Williams and colleagues[25] looked at conditions reported when screening 297 people aged over 75 years, and examined whether the diagnoses were previously known or not. Problems reaching the 1% level of prevalence and previously undiagnosed included hearing loss, cataracts, total cancers, hypertension, diabetes mellitus, varicose veins/ulcers and anaemia. Previously diagnosed problems where treatment could be improved included dementia, depression, foot disabilities, locomotor problems, obesity and glaucoma.

Anderson's 1976 classification of three areas of preventive care in the elderly – physical, mental and social – remains useful, although in practice these areas are very closely interrelated and one often impinges on another.[26]

Anderson also made the important point, reinforced recently by the Royal Commission on Long-Term Care, that elderly people are ill not because they are old but because there is something wrong with them.

Physical screening

In their authoritative review of screening in the elderly, Bulpitt and colleagues[24] looked at 13 possible screening tests evaluated on the basis of 10 criteria. They suggested that screening may be worthwhile with regard to need for chiropody and for varicose veins/ulcer, hearing loss, obesity, visual impairment, hypothyroidism, hypertension, anaemia and diabetes mellitus. However, they stressed that these assessments need to be tested prospectively in randomised controlled trials.

Hypertension

Blood pressure should be measured regularly in patients over 60 years of age, since risk of morbidity from hypertension is known to increase with age. Results from a number of randomised controlled trials[27–32] have shown that treatment for hypertension is beneficial in reducing rates of stroke, coronary artery disease and death. Earlier recommendations stressed the value of screening for hypertension in middle age, but there is now good evidence for extending these recommendations to individuals over 65 years of age. Signs of early heart failure could also be identified by asking about undue shortness of breath.

Patterson and Logan[33] state that hypertension affects at least 10% of people over the age of 65 years, and 20% of those over the age of 80 years. They recommend that case finding should be considered in those aged 65–84 years, and that individual clinical judgement should be exercised when considering treatment. Unanswered questions include the efficacy of treatment for hypertension in patients over the age of 80 years, the effects of medication on quality of life, and possible side-effects, particularly in those who have other coexisting diseases.

Hearing loss

Hearing impairment is common in people over 60 years of age.[34] Age-related hearing loss usually develops gradually over a number of years, and a significant proportion of those affected may not be aware of the problem, although it can have adverse consequences for quality of life and effective communication and social functioning.

The US Preventive Services Task Force recommends that older adults should be screened by periodic questioning about their hearing and making referrals where appropriate.[35] As Patterson[36] has pointed out, screening in the form of a single question and use of an audioscope can be performed easily in the primary care setting, and referral for full audiological examination can be made if necessary.

Sight

As with hearing loss, problems with sight can have a significant effect on the functions of daily living, and poor vision is considered to be a common unreported condition in the elderly population. For example, Reinstein and colleagues[37] found that 34% of an elderly population in England had functionally significant correctable undetected visual acuity deficit in one or both eyes. In contrast, Keane and colleagues,[38] in a study of eye screening of an elderly community-based population in Ireland, showed a relatively low prevalence of correctable undetected eye defects (only 8.6% of those studied required referral for further management). However, these authors recommended that routine assessment of elderly patients should include screening of visual acuity, since subjects are apt to overestimate the adequacy of their vision. They cite a study of 202 subjects which found that although only 34 individuals reported inadequate vision, 72 were found to have significant visual impairment.

Smeeth and Iliffe[39] conducted a systematic review of randomised controlled trials of population screening in the community that included any assessment of vision or visual function with at least 6 months of follow-up. They found outcome data on vision for 3494 people in five trials of multi-phasic assessment. Evidence for the effectiveness of visual screening was lacking, but they could not exclude a small beneficial effect. In a later study to determine the effect of screening for visual impairment in those aged over 75 years in general practice, Smeeth and colleagues[40] found that a vision screen component performed by a practice nurse did not improve visual outcome.

Patterson[41] points out that visual loss can be detected readily with a sight card, and that correction of refractive errors and surgery for cataract lead to an improvement in quality of life. He suggests that there is fair evidence for including screening with the Snellen sight card in any periodic health examination of the elderly. Individuals at risk of developing glaucoma (e.g. those with diabetes or a positive family history) should undergo periodic assessment by an ophthalmologist.

In 1996 the US Preventive Services Task Force stated that there was insufficient evidence to argue for or against routine screening for intra-ocular hypertension or glaucoma in primary care, but that high-risk patients should be sent for evaluation by an eye specialist.[35]

The report of an American study in 2002, *Vision Problems in the US*, concluded that loss of sight in the ageing population was becoming a source of great concern.[42,43] The main investigator, David Friedman, saw the report as a 'wake-up call to the need for better screening and treatment of preventable vision loss.' The four main causes of loss of eyesight, namely diabetic retinopathy, age-related macular degeneration, cataract and glaucoma, can all be treated to some extent if they are detected early enough, but this is not happening. The US findings are applicable to all developed countries, and screening, early detection and prompt intervention could contribute significantly to controlling problems with sight as the population ages.

Asymptomatic and previously undetected conditions

The prevalence of asymptomatic bacteriuria increases with age and is known to be higher in institutionalised populations. However, it is not associated with increased mortality and there is currently insufficient evidence to recommend routine screening.[44]

De Craen and colleagues[45] reported a study that assessed the number of previously known and newly identified patients with anaemia, diabetes mellitus, thyroid dysfunction, atrial fibrillation and hypertension in a population-based sample of 85-year-old individuals. Using information from GP and pharmacy records combined with five simple and readily available procedures, they obtained estimates of the prevalence of these five common clinical abnormalities.

There were a considerable number of people with previously undetected anaemia and hypertension, but fewer with the other three abnormalities. They assert that it is feasible to use these investigative procedures in an elderly population in order to provide important quantitative information for future discussions on screening for the elderly.

However, there are clear practical arguments against this sort of approach in the very elderly. De Craen's paper generated a response from one general practitioner who made the point that treating those previously undiagnosed with diabetes, hypertension and atrial fibrillation with aspirin and warfarin would result in more anaemia. Acknowledging his risk of being considered paternalistic and out of touch, he also said 'I sometimes think there should be a moratorium on investigating the asymptomatic over-85s – most of whom would prefer to be left alone.'

Incontinence

Urinary incontinence is reported to affect 15–39% of the over-65s living in the community.[46] If left untreated, it is an unpleasant and socially embarrassing condition that increases the risk of infection, social isolation and depression. Effective treatment is available, and improvement can be achieved for most individuals if the problem is identified. Screening can be performed by discreet questioning in a routine surgery visit, but this is an extremely sensitive area and some patients may resent such perceived intrusion.

Lack of physical activity

Lack of regular physical activity is a major and unrecognised risk factor for disability in older adults, and the Report of the HMO Care Management Workgroup in the USA recommends a programme of regular activity and exercise even in those who are relatively frail.[47]

Certainly in the UK there has been a recent increase in awareness of the benefits of physical activity, and in local authority and private provision for this at all ages.

Foot problems

Allied to physical activity, assessment of foot problems and provision of chiropody represent another area that can make a huge difference in improving mobility and helping older people to remain active and independent.[48] However, Bulpitt and colleagues[24] point out that in this context it is essential to consider whether the present healthcare system and the chiropody services in particular would be willing and able to cope with the large numbers of elderly people involved, most of whom would need this service to deal with common treatable problems such as ulcers, ingrowing toenails and athlete's foot.

Harvey and colleagues drew attention to this problem in a population-based study of foot morbidity and exposure to chiropody.[49] They found that although one-third of pensioners received chiropody, the NHS gives low priority to foot problems and chiropody is regarded as a low-status service. They suggested that consideration should be given to ways of identifying individuals with severe foot morbidity and of providing accessible services.

Inappropriate medication

A study by the US Agency for Healthcare Research and Quality (AHRQ) in 2001 highlighted the problem of inappropriate medication in elderly patients in the USA.[50]

According to the findings, about 20% of the approximately 32 million elderly Americans living in the community in 1996 used at least one or more of 33 prescription medicines considered to be potentially inappropriate. Nearly one million elderly patients used at least one of 11 medicines which a panel of geriatric medicine and pharmacy experts advising the researchers agreed should always be avoided in the elderly. These included long-acting benzodiazepines, sedative or hypnotic drugs, analgesics and anti-emetics.

The Report of the HMO Care Management Workgroup also highlighted this problem, and estimated that approximately 14–24% of community-based older adults take medication that is believed to be inappropriate.[51]

A system of regular surveillance of the elderly in primary care should certainly include a review of the current medication of individual patients, with clear and specific guidance targeted at healthcare professionals and the public.

Mental health screening

The two main problems in this area are depression and dementia.

Depression

Depression is a common but frequently unrecognised or inadequately treated condition in the elderly population.[52] However, if properly diagnosed, there are effective treatments available for severe depression. Mild to moderate depression may respond to efforts to reduce social isolation without the need for medication.

In 1996, the US Preventive Services Task Force found insufficient evidence to support or rule out routine screening for depression. However, in an update of its position in 2002 it urged that doctors should routinely screen all adult patients for the condition.[53]

Watson and Pignone[54] conducted a systematic review of the accuracy of depression screening instruments for older adults in primary care. They concluded that accurate and feasible instruments are available for diagnosis, although more research is needed to determine the accuracy of depression screening for individuals with dementia.

Hope[55] is among those who have highlighted the important role of the community nurse in identifying depression in the elderly and providing an appropriate response.

In a randomised controlled trial of a large and diverse population of older adults with arthritis and comorbid depression, Lin and colleagues[56] found that the benefits of improving depression care extended beyond reducing depressive symptoms and included decreased pain as well as improved functional status and quality of life.

A recent American study of depression and comorbid illnesses in elderly primary care patients found that treating depression in primary care can improve patients' quality of life despite other illnesses.[57] Depression in this age group is often considered to be related to physical illness, but it can also arise from life events and circumstances such as the death of a spouse, retirement, social isolation and reduced income. These authors contend that 'treatment for depression can lead to more dramatic improvements in functional status, disability, and quality of life than interventions for other chronic illnesses.'

Dementia

The prevalence of severe dementia in people aged 65 years or over in the community is between 2.5% and 5.0%,[58] and there is currently no effective treatment for most of those affected. Alzheimer's disease is the commonest cause, but infections, metabolic disturbances and drug-induced side-effects can also cause or exacerbate mental confusion. Depression may also occasionally mimic dementia.

Palmer and colleagues[59] reported a community study to evaluate a simple three-step procedure for identifying pre-clinical Alzheimer's disease and dementia in the general population. They concluded that although the measure used had a high positive predictive value (dependent on reporting memory loss), it only identified 18% of those who subsequently developed dementia.

Early diagnosis can be helpful in allowing time to plan for subsequent deterioration. However, the harm caused by labelling an individual as demented must be weighed against any possible benefits, particularly when dealing with dementias that are potentially reversible.

In 1996, the US Preventive Services Task Force recommended against screening for dementia.[35] In an update in 2003,[60] they again concluded that there is insufficient evidence to argue for or against screening in older adults, and that there is a need for further research to determine whether any benefits from screening outweigh the potential harms. They found evidence that some screening tests have good sensitivity but only fair specificity in detecting cognitive impairment and dementia. And although a number of drug treatments appear to delay the natural progression of Alzheimer's disease very slightly, it is far from clear whether the modest benefits observed in drug trials can be generalised to patients detected in routine primary care.

Patterson, in his report for the Canadian Task Force,[58] also found insufficient evidence to argue for or against screening. He stated that further trials of screening are needed to examine the impact of detection of cognitive impairment, its subsequent investigation and treatment. Studies should also be directed towards discovering any negative effects associated with attaching the labels of Alzheimer's disease or cognitive impairment to an individual. He concludes:

> Despite the theoretical advantages of identifying individuals with cognitive impairment, there is no evidence to suggest whether this leads to a net benefit or risk to the individual. Although pharmaceutical agents are able to produce measurable changes in cognitive performance in people with Alzheimer's disease, none has been shown to result consistently in clinically significant improvement.[58]

Alcohol-related problems

O'Connell and colleagues[61] looked at alcohol use disorders in elderly people, and concluded that they are common and associated with considerable morbidity. They are also liable to be under-detected and misdiagnosed for various reasons, and the recommended limits for intake, appropriate screening instruments and diagnostic criteria should be redefined for elderly people.

In an American study of the use of alcohol by community-based older adults, Resnick and colleagues[62] suggested that healthcare providers should use an individualised approach and help individuals to establish safe drinking habits that will improve their health and quality of life.

Social screening

Home visits

This area of assessment is likely to devolve more on the health visitor/community nurse and social worker than on the general practitioner. Home circumstances and family and social networks are a vital part of any support system for the elderly. Knowledge of these can provide useful information on the need for home visits, medical care, home helps, meals on wheels and day-care centres, and this can help to improve quality of life in this age group.

The study of home visits to patients over 75 years of age over a three-year period by Hendriksen and colleagues,[6] mentioned earlier in the chapter, found that preventive visiting is a feasible way for the community to meet the demands of elderly people who want to stay in their own homes for as long as possible. However, for this method to work they state that 'one person should coordinate the programme, be available every day, have a thorough knowledge of social and medical systems, and have an understanding and devoted interest in elderly people.'

Also as mentioned earlier, Clark[3] contends that the effectiveness of preventive home visits to the elderly cannot be judged properly by randomised controlled trials. She warns that 'The lack of a clear justification for preventive home visits to older people, in terms of the outcomes of mortality, institutionalisation and particular measures of function, should not be used as an excuse for discontinuing the service.'

Elkan and colleagues conducted a systematic review and meta-analysis of home-based support for older people.[63] Their outcome measures were mortality, admission to hospital, admission to institutional care, functional status and health status. They found that home-visiting care was associated with a significant reduction in mortality and in admission to long-term institutional care. In view of the conflicting results from the studies included in their analysis, they suggest that future studies would benefit from a greater focus on the process of delivery of care and on attempting to identify which components of the intervention work well and which populations benefit most.

They support the view that health visitors are well placed to promote the health of older people and to provide surveillance and support. Historically, British health visitors have provided services mainly to mothers and young children but, with current demographic changes, there is surely considerable potential for increasing their role in working with older people in the community. There is anecdotal evidence that this is already happening, with health visitors in some areas taking responsibility for the initial assessment of the over-75s and referring those in need of medical attention to general practitioners. There may be a resource implication here that would need to be addressed.

Falls

The Canadian Preventive Services Task Force found insufficient evidence to support the inclusion of assessment and counselling in the routine health examination of the elderly.[64] After a fall that has caused injury, assessment of balance and gait might usefully be carried out and information provided on the use of safety features in the home.

More than 30% of older adults in the community fall at least once a year, and 50% do so more than once. The Report of the HMO Care Management Work-group stresses the importance of intervention in those who are at high risk for future falls, most of whom can be identified by a simple screening question about the number of falls during a six-month period. They claim that multiple falls are a marker of physical frailty, since falls and fear of falling frequently lead to reduced activity, social isolation and consequently impaired function.[65] Practical treatment options in this area include exercise classes and hip protectors.

Under-nutrition

The HMO group have also drawn attention to the problem of under-nutrition and state that as many as 15% of older adults in the community suffer from inadequate nutrition, about half of whom are unrecognised and therefore untreated. There are many contributing factors here. It may be difficult for older people to get to the shops, financial resources may be limited, and those whose partners and children have died or moved away may not have the motivation to cook properly for themselves. The HMO group recommends that body weight should be measured at every surgery visit and any individual who has lost 10 pounds or more over the previous six months should receive further assessment.[66]

Elder abuse

Elder abuse is being increasingly recognised as a significant health and social problem, particularly at present in North America. Its scope and definition currently lack precise boundaries, tools for screening are not well evaluated and there is no clear evidence that interventions are effective. The Canadian Preventive Services Task Force has concluded that there is insufficient evidence for or against covering this in a periodic health examination, but there are a numbered of unanswered questions that should be priorities for research.[67]

Summary and conclusions

Society is facing a major challenge with regard to how best to maintain health and quality of life in a population where the number of people aged over 60 years now exceeds the number aged under 16 years.

Table 7.4 Our recommendations for assessment of the elderly in primary care

Physical assessment	Mental assessment	Social assessment
Hypertension	Depression	Falls
Early heart failure	Alcohol use	Under-nutrition
Hearing loss		Isolation
Vision loss		
Incontinence		
Lack of physical activity		
Foot problems		
Review of medication		

A system of regular surveillance and case finding in primary care would seem to be the most appropriate form of screening, particularly in individuals aged 75 years or over, but the resource implications of this for general practice must be confronted. Several simple tests, such as identifying difficulties with sight or hearing or problems with feet, can make a huge difference to comfort and quality of life. Depression is another area in which identification and treatment could improve well-being. Social and community support are also vital in enabling older people to enjoy as independent and contented a life as possible.

Our recommendations for assessment of the elderly in primary care are summarised in Table 7.4.

Launching a campaign to ensure that older people are treated with dignity in Britain's hospitals, the *Observer* newspaper stated that 'The good society cannot allow the old to become disposable commodities living at the margins . . . it is in all our interests to promote the dignity and self-respect of the elderly.' The emphasis in screening for this age group should be on improving quality of life and preserving function and independence, rather than on providing heroic treatments to prevent mortality.

References

1 www.statistics.gov.uk/census2001

2 Royal Commission on Long-Term Care (1999) *With Respect to Old Age. Long-term care – rights and responsibilities.* Cm.4192–1 (Chairman, Sir Stewart Sutherland). The Stationery Office, London.

3 Clark J (2001) Preventive home visits to elderly people (editorial). *BMJ.* **323**: 708.

4 Freedman GR, Charlewood JE and Dodds PA (1978) Screening the aged in general practice. *J R Coll Gen Pract.* **28**: 421–5.

5 Tulloch AJ and Moore V (1979) A randomised controlled trial of geriatric screening and surveillance in general practice. *J R Coll Gen Pract.* **29**: 733–42.

6 Hendriksen C, Lund E and Stromgard E (1984) Consequences of assessment and intervention among elderly people: a three-year randomised controlled trial. *BMJ.* **289**: 1522–4.

7 Hendriksen C, Lund E and Stromgard E (1989) Hospitalisation of elderly people: a three-year controlled trial. *J Am Geriatr Soc.* **37**: 117–22.

8 Khaw KT, Reeve J, Luben R *et al.* (2004) Quantitative ultrasonography of the calcaneus

predicts total and hip fractures in men and women: the EPIC-Norfolk prospective population study. *Lancet.* **363**: 197–202.

9 Trivedi D and Khaw KT (2001) Dehydroepiandrosterone sulphate and mortality in elderly men and women. *J Clin Epidemiol Metab.* **86**: 4171–7.

10 Trivedi D, Doll R and Khaw KT (2003) Randomised double-blind controlled trial of four-monthly vitamin D supplementation on fractures and mortality in men and women. *BMJ.* **326**: 469–72.

11 Department of Health (2001) *The National Service Framework for Older People.* The Stationery Office, London.

12 Health Departments of Great Britain (1989) *General Practice in the National Health Service: the 1990 Contract.* Department of Health, London.

13 www.doh.gov.uk/gmscontract (April 2004).

14 Freer CB (1985) Geriatric screening: a reappraisal of preventive strategies in the care of the elderly. *J R Coll Gen Pract.* **35**: 288–90.

15 Williams ES and Barley NH (1985) Old people not known to the general practitioner: low-risk group. *BMJ.* **291**: 251–4.

16 National Statistics (2000) *Living in Britain;* www.statistics.gov.uklib/viewerChart260.html

17 National Statistics (2000) *Living in Britain;* www.statistics.gov.uklib/viewerChart287.html

18 Buckley EG and Williamson J (1988) What sort of 'health checks' for older people? *BMJ.* **296**: 1144–5.

19 Freer CB (1987) Consultation-based screening of the elderly in general practice: a pilot study. *J R Coll Gen Pract.* **37**: 455–6.

20 Van Haastregt JCM, Diederiks JPM, van Rossum E, de Witte LP and Crebolder HFJM (2000) Effects of preventive home visits to elderly people living in the community: systematic review. *BMJ.* **320**: 754–8.

21 Smeeth L, Fletcher AE, Stirling S *et al.* (2001) Randomised comparison of three methods of administering a screening questionnaire to elderly people: findings from the MRC trial of the assessment and management of older people in the community. *BMJ.* **323**: 1403–7.

22 Thomson H, Hoskins R, Petticrew M *et al.* (2004) Evaluating the health effects of social interventions. *BMJ.* **328**: 283–5.

23 Williamson J, Stokoe IH, Gray S *et al.* (1964) Old people at home. Their unreported needs. *Lancet.* **i**: 1117–20.

24 Bulpitt CJ, Benos AS, Nicoll CG and Fletcher AE (1990) Should medical screening for the elderly population be promoted? *Gerontology.* **36**: 230–45.

25 Williams EI, Bennett FM, Nixon JV *et al.* (1972) Socio-medical study of patients over 75 in general practice. *BMJ.* **ii**: 445–8.

26 Anderson WF (1979) Preventive medicine in the elderly. In: K Hazell (ed.) *Social and Medical Problems of the Elderly* (4e). Hutchison, London.

27 Amery A, Birkenhager W, Brixko P *et al.* (1985) Mortality and morbidity results from the European Working Party on High Blood Pressure in the Elderly Trial. *Lancet.* **1**: 1349–54.

28 Amery A, Birkenhager W, Brixko P *et al.* (1986) Efficacy of antihypertensive drug treatment according to age, sex, blood pressure and previous cardiovascular disease in patients over the age of 60. *Lancet.* **2**: 589–92.

29 Staessan J, Bulpitt C, Clement D *et al.* (1989) Relation between mortality and treated blood pressure in elderly people with hypertension: report of the European Working Party on High Blood Pressure in the Elderly. *BMJ.* **298**: 1552–6.

30 SHEP Cooperative Research Group (1991) Prevention of stroke by antihypertensive drug treatment in older persons with isolated systolic hypertension. *JAMA.* **265**: 3255–64.

31 Vogt TM, Ireland CC, Black D *et al.* (1986) Recruitment of elderly volunteers for multi-centre clinical trials: the SHEO pilot study. *Control Clin Trials.* **7**: 118–23.

32 Hypertension Detection Follow-up Cooperative Group (1979) Five-year findings of the Hypertension Detection Follow-up Program. *JAMA.* **242**: 2562–77.

33 Patterson C and Logan AG (2003) Hypertension in the elderly: case finding and treatment to prevent vascular disease. In: *The Canadian Guide to Clinical Preventive Health Care*; www.hcsc.gc.ca/hppb/healthcare/pubs/clinical_preventive/sec11e.htm

34 Davis AC (1991) Epidemiological profile of hearing impairments: the scale and nature of the problem with special reference to the elderly. *Acta Otolaryngol Suppl Stockh.* **476**: 23–31.

35 US Preventive Services Task Force (1996) *Guide to Clinical Preventive Services* (2e); www.ahrq.gov/clinic/prevenix.htm

36 Patterson C (2003) Prevention of hearing impairment and disability in the elderly. In: *The Canadian Guide to Clinical Preventive Health Care*; www.hcsc.gc.ca/hppb/healthcare/pubs/clinical_preventive/sec11e.htm

37 Reinstein DZ, Dorward NL, Wormald RP *et al.* (1993) Correctable undetected visual acuity deficit in patients aged 65 and over attending an Accident and Emergency Department. *Br J Ophthalmol.* **77**: 293–6.

38 Keane E, Coakley D, Walsh JB and Connor MO (1997) Eye screening in the elderly. *Ir Med J.* **90**. Online article.

39 Smeeth L and Iliffe S (1998) Effectiveness of screening older people for impaired vision in a community setting: systematic review of evidence from randomised controlled trials. *BMJ.* **316**: 660–63.

40 Smeeth L, Fletcher AE, Hanciles S, Evans J and Wormald R (2003) Screening older people for impaired vision in primary care: cluster randomised trial. *BMJ.* **327**: 1027.

41 Patterson C (2003) Screening for visual impairment in the elderly. In: *The Canadian Guide to Clinical Preventive Health Care*; www.hcsc.gc.ca/hppb/healthcare/pubs/clinical_preventive/sec11e.htm

42 Senior K (2002) Vision problems in the US. Report of a 2001 Consensus Meeting (news report). *Lancet.* **359**: 1129.

43 National Institutes of Health (2002) *Vision Problems in the US: prevalence of adult vision impairment and age-related eye disease in America*; www.nei.nih.gov/eyedata

44 Nicolle LE (2003) Screening for asymptomatic bacteriuria in the elderly. In: *The Canadian Guide to Clinical Preventive Health Care*; www.hcsc.gc.ca/hppb/healthcare/pubs/clinical_preventive/sec11e.htm

45 De Craen AJM, Gussekloo J, Teng YKO, Macfarlane P and Westendorp RGJ (2003) Prevalence of five common clinical abnormalities in very elderly people: population-based cross-sectional study. *BMJ.* **327**: 131–2.

46 HMO Workgroup on Care Management (2002) Urinary incontinence. In: *Improving the Care of Older Adults with Common Geriatric Conditions*. American Association of Health Plans Foundation, Washington, DC.

47 HMO Workgroup on Care Management (2002) Physical inactivity. In: *Improving the Care of Older Adults with Common Geriatric Conditions*. American Association of Health Plans Foundation, Washington, DC.

48 Helfand AE (2003) Podiatric assessment of the geriatric patient. *Clin Podiatr Med Surg.* **20**: 407–29.

49 Harvey I, Frankel S, Marks R, Shalom D and Morgan M (1997) Foot morbidity and exposure to chiropody: population-based study. *BMJ.* **315**: 1054–5.

50 Zhan C, Sangl J, Bierman AS *et al.* (2001) Potentially inappropriate medication use in the community-dwelling elderly: findings from the 1996 Medical Expenditure Panel Survey. *JAMA.* **286**: 2823–9.

51 HMO Workgroup on Care Management (2002) Medication-related complications. In: *Improving the Care of Older Adults with Common Geriatric Conditions*. American Association of Health Plans Foundation, Washington, DC.

52 Lapid MI and Rummans TA (2003) Evaluation and management of geriatric depression in primary care. *Mayo Clin Proc.* **78**: 423–9.

53 US Preventive Services Task Force (2002) *Guide to Clinical Preventive Services* (2e); www.ahcpr.gov/clinic/uspstfix.htm

54 Watson LC and Pignone MP (2003) Screening accuracy for late-life depression in primary care: a systematic review. *J Fam Pract.* **52**: 956–64.

55 Hope K (2003) A hidden problem: identifying depression in older people. *Br J Commun Nurs.* **8**: 314–20.

56 Linn EHB, Katon W, Von Korff M *et al.* (2003) Effect of improving depression care on pain and functional outcomes among older adults with arthritis. *JAMA.* **290**: 2428–34.

57 Hitchcock Noel P, Williams JW Jr, Unutzer J *et al.* (2004) Depression and comorbid illness in elderly primary care patients: impact on multiple domains of health status and well-being. *Ann Fam Med.* **2**: 555–62.

58 Patterson C (2003) Screening for cognitive impairment in the elderly. In: *The Canadian Guide to Clinical Preventive Health Care*; www.hcsc.gc.ca/hppb/healthcare/pubs/clinical_preventive/sec11c75.htm

59 Palmer K, Backman L, Winblad B and Fratiglioni L (2003) Detection of Alzheimer's disease and dementia in the pre-clinical phase: population-based cohort study. *BMJ.* **326**: 245–50.

60 US Preventive Services Task Force (1996, update 2003) *Guide to Clinical Preventive Services* (2e); www.ahrq.gov/clinic/prevenix.htm

61 O'Connell H, Chin A-V, Cunningham C and Lawlor B (2003) Alcohol use disorders in elderly people – redefining an age-old problem in old age. *BMJ.* **327**: 664–7.

62 Resnick B, Perry D, Applebaum G *et al.* (2003) The impact of alcohol use in community-dwelling older adults. *J Commun Health Nurs.* **20**: 135–45.

63 Elkan R, Kendrick D, Dewey M *et al.* (2001) Effectiveness of home-based support for older people: systematic review and meta-analysis. *BMJ.* **323**: 719–24.

64 Elford RW (2003) Prevention of household and recreational injuries in the elderly. In: *The Canadian Guide to Clinical Preventive Health Care*; www.hcsc.gc.ca/hppb/healthcare/pubs/clinical_preventive/sec11c75.htm

65 HMO Workgroup on Care Management (2002) Falls. In: *Improving the Care of Older Adults with Common Geriatric Conditions*. American Association of Health Plans Foundation, Washington, DC.

66 HMO Workgroup on Care Management (2002) Under-nutrition. In: *Improving the Care of Older Adults with Common Geriatric Conditions*. American Association of Health Plans Foundation, Washington, DC.

67 Patterson C (2003) Secondary prevention of elder abuse. In: *The Canadian Guide to Clinical Preventive Health Care*; www.hcsc.gc.ca/hppb/healthcare/pubs/clinical_preventive/sec11c75.htm.

Chapter 8

Screening practices in Europe*

One of the key questions is whether screening tests reflect a patholo-
gisation of many healthy people or whether, on the contrary, they
reflect a good service offered to a few sick people, and one that can also
be reassuring for the healthy subjects being examined.†

Introduction

In order to determine screening practice in Europe we looked at screening in six
countries, namely Italy, Spain, Sweden, Denmark, Germany and France. These
illustrate a variety of different approaches to health service provision and
financing. In each case a key informant was identified and was extremely helpful
in providing us with details. We asked each informant whether the country in
question had a national policy on screening and whether an official body was
responsible for the formulation of policy, what screening tests were recommended and reimbursed, what mechanisms existed for ensuring that appropriate
groups were included and tested, whether there were non-professional pressures
to introduce (or discontinue) screening programmes, and who was responsible for
treatment or further investigation if an abnormality was found at screening.

The countries chosen have widely different healthcare systems. Italy has a
national health service similar in structure and organisation to that in the UK.
Spain also has a national health service, but with major devolution of power to
regional levels. Sweden and Denmark have national health services with
financing for specific services at local levels. France and Germany each have a
universal social health insurance system, although the administrative methods
differ. Beyond this summary, we do not consider it appropriate to detail each
health system except where it impacts on screening policy and practice.

Italy

There is no national screening body equivalent to our own UK National Screening
Committee. However, screening practice is very similar to that in the UK, with the
addition of screening for colorectal cancer, which is recommended and is already
performed regularly.

Spain

Screening activities are the responsibility of regional governments. As an illus-
tration of this, the policies and procedures in the Valencian community (one of

* We are grateful to the following who provided information for this chapter: M Brodin,
D Delnoy, N Klazinga, E Lynge, M McKee, M Rosen, L Salas, F Schelp and N Segnan.
† Danish Council of Ethics (2001) *Screening: a report*. Danish Council of Ethics, Copenhagen.

the 17 regions) will be described. This region has a population of about four million inhabitants and has a hospital network distributed throughout the different health areas. These hospitals are responsible for follow-up and treatment of any abnormalities identified.

There is a breast cancer screening programme and also a screening programme for cervical cancer. Screening activities are supervised by representatives of epidemiology, surgery and oncology, medical physics, radiology and health administration. Breast cancer screening is a population-based service for women aged 45–69 years, who are invited for screening at two-yearly intervals. Positive cases are referred to a reference hospital, which can be either in the public network or in a private state-assisted hospital. Cervical cancer screening by Pap smear is carried out on women aged 25–65 years who attend the health service – that is, it is opportunistic. The recommended interval between tests is three years.

There are considered to be insufficient grounds to screen for any other cancers at present, although piloting for colorectal cancer has begun.

Sweden

Sweden has a national health service with a great deal of devolution, in terms of finance and authority, to local government.

There is no national screening policy, but recommendations and guidance are given for specific procedures. The official body responsible for this is the National Board of Health and Welfare. This is advised by the Swedish Council on Technology Assessment in Health Care (SBU), which reviews and synthesises published literature on different medical technologies.

Opinion in Sweden is sceptical of the value of 'general screening.' This is despite – or perhaps because of – the Varmland experiment carried out by the Jungners in the 1960s in which the population underwent a biochemical screen with little benefit. A number of specified criteria need to be fulfilled before recommendations are made for screening for specific conditions. These are similar to the commonly accepted criteria discussed in Chapter 1.

There are national recommendations for breast and cervical screening. The responsibility for these lies with the County Councils, which have final control. The age groups included and the recommended intervals for screening differ between Counties. Quality indicators for these services have been recommended, such as the proportion of women attending (of those invited) by age, recall response, severity of cases detected (stage distribution) and number of cancers detected between the regular screening tests (interval cancers). Several (but not all) centres have implemented checks for quality control. A national quality register for cervical cancer has been established, and there is a plan for a similar register for mammography.

The major pressure for screening is from the medical profession, not from the public, particularly for prostate and colorectal cancers. The SBU has recently concluded that there is no evidence for recommending screening for prostate cancer, although there may be a case for colorectal cancer screening. The Federation of County Councils is currently discussing the feasibility of this.

Denmark

Denmark has a national health system, and recommendations on screening are provided by the Danish National Board of Health. It is up to the individual counties (of which there are 15 in total) to decide on implementation.

It is recommended that Pap smears be offered every three years to women aged 23–59 years, and this is done in 14 counties. In one county, only women aged 25–45 years are included. Most positive Pap smears are referred to the local county hospitals for colposcopy in outpatient clinics, and in some areas private gynaecologists have agreements with the national health insurance to undertake these examinations.

Although there is a law which requires all counties to offer mammography screening, there is no date set by which this has to be implemented. At present the recommendation is that it should be performed every second year in women aged 50–69 years. So far only two counties have implemented this. In each of these, all assessments and any surgery are performed within one hospital. Women are invited individually to undergo the tests, and two reminders are sent in the event of non-attendance. Women can ask to be excluded from screening.

A variety of expert committees review which screening tests should be done. So far only mammography and Pap smears are recommended, although within Denmark mammography screening has been the subject of vigorous public debate. Lung specialists have put forward proposals for a randomised controlled trial of low-dose CT scanning for lung cancer. A pilot scheme for faecal occult blood testing has been recommended but has not yet been implemented.

Germany*

Germany has a national health insurance system but there is no national body responsible for screening policy. Legislation allows insured individuals to have what is known as 'early diagnosis' for cancers of the cervix, colon, breast, prostate, skin and kidney and also for certain metabolic and cardiovascular risk factors and diseases, such as blood pressure and cholesterol levels, diabetes, gout, proteinuria and 'arteriosclerosis of the heart, brain and limbs.'

It is important to recognise that although the Wilson–Jungner principles have been accepted in Germany, screening is not population based and is dependent on individuals requesting the examination. About 14% of adult men and 54% of adult women undergo screening (early-diagnosis) examinations annually.

Mammography has been the subject of heated discourse in medical journals, medical giveaway publications and the popular press. The Federal Health Ministry as well as the Association of Insurance Doctors are very much in favour of it.

Antenatal (after week 13 of pregnancy) and postnatal examinations are performed and reimbursed, and in childhood examinations for abnormalities up to the age of 6 years are also reimbursed.

---

* Full details of screening practice in Germany are described by Abholz HH (1991) In: TH Elkeles *et al.* (eds) *Prävention und Prophylaxe*. Sigma, Berlin.

France

France has a national system of health insurance and no one national body is responsible for screening. The Direction Générale de la Santé has general responsibility for health services, including screening. Specific rules for reimbursement exist for diabetes and some forms of cancer from the Securité Sociale. The local health authorities (Collectivitiés Territoriales) are responsible for the implementation of screening for the mother and child and for cancers, and education authorities (Education Nationale) are responsible for screening in teenagers. INSERM (equivalent to the MRC) has five research units working on a number of screening issues.

Conclusion

Although all of the countries questioned have accepted the need for stringent principles for screening for disease, only Sweden outside the UK has a single national body for reviewing tests and practice. Population-based screening is limited to Spain, Sweden and Denmark. In those countries that have a social insurance system, screening is based on demand (facultative, opportunistic), although it is reimbursed in all. Formalisation of quality control, further investigation and treatment is present in Spain, Sweden and Denmark to a greater or lesser extent.

Germany appears to have the most vociferous lobbies for screening, while Denmark and Sweden are relatively controlled and under little pressure to introduce new services.

Despite all of the current criticisms of the National Health Service, the structure and performance of screening services in the UK could serve as a model for other countries.

Chapter 9

Overview and recommendations

There is an ethical difference between everyday medical practice and screening. If a patient asks a medical practitioner for help, the doctor does the best he can. He is not responsible for defects in medical knowledge. If, however, the practitioner initiates screening procedures, he is in a very different situation. He should have conclusive evidence that screening can alter the natural history of the disease in a significant proportion of those screened.*

Introduction

A superficial look at screening and screening policies in the UK might point to the conclusion that little has changed since the publication of our previous book in 1990. The principles first accepted in 1968 continue to govern the policies, with some minor modifications.

Remarkably few new screening procedures have satisfied the established criteria and been introduced. Although the literature on currently accepted tests has expanded greatly with many more substantive reviews, little that is new has emerged on subjects such as cancer screening. Some aspects are still controversial.

However, some things have changed. The organisation and coordination of screening have undoubtedly improved, but perhaps the most striking change has been a shift in attitudes, both on the part of healthcare professionals and among the public.

Around 15 to 20 years ago, the medical profession was in general in favour of developing and implementing screening practice for a wide variety of conditions. The distinction between normal clinical practice and screening, first put forward by Cochrane and Holland, and quoted above, was not generally accepted. In this regard the situation has changed greatly. Doctors have now accepted that before screening for any condition is introduced, effective means of treatment and follow-up and the resources for this have to be in place. There is now much greater professional emphasis on assessing the possible harmful effects of screening as well as the benefits, and a much more considered attitude on the part of those responsible for screening policies.

The public and its political representatives, on the other hand, appear to view screening as a panacea and have great difficulty in understanding its limitations or the harm it can do. The reality – that when thousands of tests are performed in a particular population, false-positive and false-negative results are inevitable – is not easy to get across, and the concept of the small yield of screening in terms of

* Cochrane AL and Holland WW (1971) Validation of screening procedures. *Br Med Bull.* 27: 3–8.

prevention of a disease (as discussed by Raffle in the context of cervical cancer[1]) is also extremely difficult to explain. One manifestation of this difficulty in effective communication has been the number of so-called scandals reported and investigated in the media, particularly in the areas of cervical cytology and mammography, where women have been wrongly diagnosed or falsely reassured.

Industry in this country has also seized on screening as a major activity. In the past, the major commercial supporters of screening were the medical insurance organisations, such as BUPA. Screening was a major money-spinner for them and could cost firms and individuals about six times more than provision of a similar service by the NHS. In addition, screening was often provided as a perk for employees and was publicised by give-away offers in newspapers and magazines. There is now even more commercial involvement in screening, in relation to both industry and medical charities. Firms that manufacture equipment for screening (e.g. for mammography), and those that produce biochemical reagents and analyse tests, as well as those that provide the necessary information technology have joined the health-screening promoters. The most extreme examples have been in Australia and the USA, as was discussed in Chapter 6. In Australia, a senior medical cancer specialist was viciously attacked for his views on prostate cancer screening by a prostate cancer charity funded by a financial services group. In the USA, the *Western Medical Journal* and its editor were vilified by a prostate cancer charity for printing an article assessing the need for prostate cancer screening. This is thought to have influenced pharmaceutical firms to withdraw their advertising from the journal.

In the UK, too, screening is in danger of becoming over-commercialised. Pressure groups promote demand for screening for conditions in which there is no evidence of benefit. Supermarket car parks are often occupied by mobile units offering screening services on payment of a fee, and pharmacies offer diagnostic kits and monitors for a variety of conditions for home use.

In this chapter we shall summarise our views on the main issues surrounding screening today, and describe what we regard as the appropriate procedures at each stage of the life cycle. We shall conclude with some thoughts on the way ahead.

General issues

As was discussed in Chapters 2 and 3, the main general issues with regard to screening today are in the areas of genetics, economics, ethics, information and audit/evaluation/quality control. They are all closely interrelated and often overlap.

Genetics

There have been huge developments in recent years with the mapping of the human genome. However, the practical results obtained from genetic screening tests have been far more limited than had been expected by their proponents. Genetic tests have precisely the same problems as other screening tests in terms of sensitivity, specificity, accuracy and validity. They do offer major advantages in a few rare conditions, as we have noted. However, although they are helpful in a few individual cases, in population terms their promise has not yet been realised.

Genetic or biochemical tests are now feasible for a large number of very rare abnormalities during the antenatal/neonatal period through tandem spectroscopy. However, diagnosis of these conditions does not satisfy screening criteria if there is no effective treatment. Protagonists maintain that the use of such tests enables parents to exercise choice and opt for termination. Yet it is unfortunate that the scientists who developed these complex and expensive tests have not yet undertaken the essential investigations of their costs as well as their benefits, and have not assessed the anxiety induced by false-positive results or the consequences of false-negative results.

Caution is essential in this area. Just because something becomes technically possible, it does not automatically become desirable. Genetic associations, as well as associations with other health-related variables, such as behaviour, can be misleading, especially in complex diseases, because association does not necessarily mean causation. Genetic tests have psychological consequences, and appropriate cost–benefit analyses must be performed before their general use.

In Chapter 2 we described the work of Vineis and colleagues[2] on some of the fundamentals of genetic screening, and the limited number of conditions to which it can usefully be applied at present. Adequate methods of quality assurance for genetic tests (and the analysis of blood spots in general) are essential, but are often forgotten in the excitement about what technology can achieve. As with other screening tests, there are considerable commercial interests at work in this field, particularly in the USA, but also increasingly in the UK.

Screening in the neonatal period for Duchenne muscular dystrophy[3] and Huntington's disease,[4] and screening for markers of late-onset conditions which may be treatable, such as polyposis coli, may become feasible in the future.

When considering such possible future developments, care must be taken to use genetic screening only for conditions for which there is a high *absolute* risk rather than a high *relative* risk. In tests that are commercially driven (e.g. the association of venous thrombosis, haemochromatosis or the presence of Apo-Enzy 4 variants for Alzheimer's disease) the relative risk may be great but the absolute risk is small.

Genetics is also a current issue in the fields of employment and occupational health. One example has been the proposed testing of occupational groups to identify those individuals who may be particularly susceptible to a specific industrial process or compound. Although this is now technically feasible, Holtzman[5] has pointed out that industry would do much more good, less expensively, by cleaning up the known, overt process or environment rather than testing workers' susceptibility to it, with all of the ethical implications that this has for confidentiality and continuing employment.

Economics

Although the application of economic principles and methods to the assessment of the value of screening for individual conditions is relatively recent, their introduction has increased the precision with which the objectives of any programme can be considered. Economic methods have also highlighted much more clearly two factors, namely opportunity costs and equity.

When cervical cancer screening was first introduced in the UK in the 1960s, few recognised that, as a result of the increased laboratory workload the programme entailed, other pathology services would be neglected. More recently, concerns have been expressed about mammography and whether the considerable expenditure on this might be more effectively directed towards an improvement in treatment services.

Work on equity has demonstrated that in some cases the disparity between those who are healthier, better educated and more affluent and those who are more deprived may be increased because the former make more use of preventive services than the latter, and thus the social gap is widened. Solutions have been suggested (e.g. only providing screening, for instance, for thalassaemia in areas with a high concentration of ethnic minority groups), but these raise important political and ethical questions.

Economic methods as applied to screening thus demonstrate how the application of social sciences can raise pertinent questions that need to be answered.

Ethics and information

As we have stated earlier, ethical issues are of great importance in the development and application of screening policy, as is the provision of balanced and understandable information for those concerned.

The fundamental ethical issue is that screening may change a healthy individual into one with concerns about some possible illness or abnormality. It is thus incumbent on those offering a screening service that effective treatment is available and provided for any abnormality which is detected or suspected. Furthermore, as we cannot overemphasise, the transaction between the individual and the service is different. Screening is proactive – the individual is approached by the service – rather than reactive. These differences are still sometimes overlooked, despite the fact that they have been accepted by most professionals for more than 30 years.

Screening services have always been an attractive proposition for business, and with the increasing involvement of private industry in the provision of health services there has been a concomitant increase in screening services provided for profit. We have already drawn attention to the increasing advertising of screening services by private groups and bodies, including single-disease medical charities, and the preoccupation with health throughout the media. To combat these pressures, it is vital that the prerequisites and limitations of screening are recognised and accepted by the public, the politicians and the media. This means that better and more convincing communication by healthcare professionals is needed.

The ethical dilemmas of screening have been addressed exhaustively both by the medical profession and by medical ethicists. For screening to be considered ethical, the following conditions must apply.

- There must be confidence about the predictive value of the test or examination.
- The practitioner must be knowledgeable about the burden of the test and whether it should be mandatory or voluntary.
- The practitioner must be knowledgeable about the course to be followed after the result is obtained (e.g. the need for further diagnostic tests and the availability and effectiveness of treatment). In all cases the individual must

be informed in language that he or she can understand about both the investigations and the treatments that may be required and their consequences.

- The situation with regard to prenatal testing must be recognised as particularly sensitive, and the value of any proposed tests must be certain. During this period the fact that, if certain abnormalities are identified, the outcome will be either a termination or the birth of a handicapped baby must also be recognised and explained to the expectant parents.

These requirements lead to the need to test empirically what information people understand in order to enable them to provide or withhold truly informed consent. Although some studies have been done, the number of rigorous evaluations that also involve implementation of good communication practice to all individuals (whether well educated or not) is sparse. We continue to neglect the importance of adequate education on such matters as risk assessment, or of tailoring the communication to the cultural and religious needs of the individual. This must also be linked to educating the healthcare professionals who administer the tests in their interpretation, consequences and effectiveness.

As was discussed in Chapter 2, the idea of informed choice is paramount and is becoming much more prominent in the screening arena. For example, Barratt and colleagues[6] recently highlighted eight issues that are critically important for the development and use of high-quality decision aids for screening. These are summarised in Box 9.1.

Box 9.1 Considerations in the development of decision aids for screening interventions, and suggestions to developers

Screening leads to over-detection and over-treatment. Present the chances of having pseudodisease as well as clinically important disease detected by screening.

Screening may include invasive follow-up investigations and treatments. Provide information about the whole of the early detection and treatment process.

The benefits of screening are delayed, whereas harms are immediate. Present balanced information about the cumulative chance of benefits and harms over equivalent time frames.

Few people experience benefits from screening compared with the number who would be expected to benefit from most treatments. Present very small numbers by using large and consistent denominators (e.g. outcomes per 1000 or per 10 000 people screened).

Individual values and preferences are critical to screening decision making. Screening decision aids need to accommodate flexibility in labelling the outcomes as benefits or harms.

The evidence base for screening decision aids is often limited. Explicitly declare where high-quality evidence is lacking; use ranges or some other method to convey uncertainty in numerical estimates.

Continued

The public attitude is that early detection and/or prevention must be good. Explain that there is a choice and the reasons why people might decide to decline screening.

Little regulation is in place to protect consumers from aggressive marketing, and there may be strong financial incentives to get people to participate in screening. Information about financial gains to the organisation that is offering the screening test may need to be included in decision aids.

Source: Barratt *et al.*[6] Reproduced with kind permission of the authors and the BMJ Publishing Group.

The concept of screening continues to pose ethical difficulties despite the superficial acceptance of the long-established principles. If an individual asks to be screened for a particular condition, there is no reason why the practitioner should not comply so long as the pros and cons are fully explained. What continues to need emphasis is that when the practitioner initiates the action – whether by inviting a population or an individual, at high or low risk, to be tested and whether this is done *de novo* or during a patient–doctor consultation for some other purpose – the ethical situation changes and screening principles must be satisfied.

Audit, evaluation and quality control

The increasing interest of the media in health service issues has had an impact on screening and screening policy. Although as with all health services there has been concern to provide a good service and to meet appropriate standards, the possibility of errors is greater than for most other procedures in healthcare. It is extremely difficult to explain and communicate the concept of false-negative and false-positive results that bedevil all screening tests. With the many thousands of tests performed in a screening programme, the likelihood of an error is not necessarily greater than for any other procedure. If one has, say, an error rate of 1 per 1000, and 1000 tests are performed per year, that error is unlikely to be noted. However, if 100 000 tests are performed, with the same error rate, 100 errors are much more likely to hit the headlines. There is therefore a need for much greater rigour in maintaining the quality control of screening. The occurrence of 'scandals' reported in the media, including errors in cervical or breast screening, is the manifestation of public concern.

The need to ensure adequate quality control of screening is well recognised, and we have outlined in Chapter 3 the various measures that need to be taken in order to ensure that quality is maintained. These are summarised again in Box 9.2 opposite.

Box 9.2 Components of adequate quality control of screening

Identification of the target population.

Identification of the individuals in the population to be screened.

Means to ensure that all those eligible for screening can attend (e.g. a personal invitation, suitable timing of screening examinations to suit the needs of those involved).

Adequate premises, equipment and staff to ensure that the screening examination is conducted under pleasant conditions and is acceptable to those attending.

An appropriate, satisfactory method of ensuring the maintenance of the best standards of the test(s) – quality assurance by:

1   initial and continuing training of the personnel performing the test(s)
2   demonstration (by appropriate records) of the maintenance standards of equipment used in the examination (e.g. calibration of X-ray machines in mammography)
3   routine checks of the validity of the tests performed (e.g. random duplicate measurements for biochemistry, cytology, and reading of X-rays).

There should be adequate and appropriate facilities for the diagnosis and treatment of any individual found to require this. There should be as little delay as possible between the screening attendance, advice that the screening test was negative, advice that the screening test result required further investigation, and referral to the appropriate centre for further investigation or treatment. A timetable should be established for these different procedures, and there should be continuous monitoring to check that the time intervals between the various stages are complied with.

There should be regular checks on the feelings of satisfaction of those who have undergone the screening process. This includes those investigated, the screen-negatives and those who were invited but who have not participated.

Finally, regular periodic checks should be made of the records of the screened individuals to ascertain their adequacy.

There is an equally pressing but under-expressed need to make the public, the media, the managers and the politicians aware of what screening is and what it is not, and why there will always be false-positive and false-negative results. With the current emphasis on the dissemination of balanced understandable information, it is crucial to ensure that individuals who are invited to undergo screening are made more aware of both the benefits and the potential harms of the procedure – and to emphasise that screening is not a universal panacea but may, like all human procedures, be fallible. It is this lack of awareness by the public, together with the inability or unwillingness of many of those administering the tests to communicate this information effectively, that represents the main failures in the process. Although most screening services have adequate systems of quality control – and audit of these – few services audit or evaluate the information exchanges between the providers and the recipients. Unless this situation is rectified, we will continue to have these so-called scandals and dissatisfaction with screening services.

Life-cycle stages

Antenatal and neonatal period

The screening tests undertaken in the antenatal and neonatal period have been discussed in detail in Chapter 4. The presence and authority of the National Screening Committee (NSC) have meant that the field is under continuous review. New tests are constantly being evaluated. We have described the situation at the time of writing, but we must emphasise that NSC recommendations are changing all the time.

The main changes over the past decade have been relatively few. The use of triple (or quadruple) screening tests combined with ultrasound measurement of nuchal thickness at first and second trimester has increased the certainty of an accurate diagnosis for Down syndrome. Gradually more and more areas in the UK are changing to this from the provision of only two tests on one occasion. Testing for cystic fibrosis has been comprehensively reviewed and recommended in a Health Technology Assessment report, and is being phased in at the neonatal stage.

The current policy on thalassaemia and sickle-cell disease screening is for the phased introduction of a programme to offer sickle-cell screening to all infants as part of the newborn bloodspot screening programme. At the antenatal stage, the plan is for the staged implementation of a programme to offer screening for sickle-cell disease and thalassaemia to all women as part of early antenatal care, starting with high-prevalence populations.

There have been few other changes at this early stage of the life cycle. Although communication between patients and doctors has undoubtedly become better in recent years, there is still scope for further improvement. The proponents of biochemical and genetic screening during the antenatal and neonatal period, for example, emphasise that it enables families to make informed choices. However, there are still major problems in the way in which information is given to the family and, most importantly, their ability to understand it. There is a need for further research on what information should be given and on patient experiences. The need to provide balanced and understandable information rather than advice has still not been fully understood by many healthcare professionals.

Childhood

With regard to screening in childhood, the only major change has been in the recommendation to screen for hearing impairment. Adequate trials have now been conducted to develop screening tests, to define the ages at which they are best applied and to develop effective methods for treatment and management.

The major ingredients now are the universal applications of screening services and treatment. One obstacle that has not been removed is the opposition of many families who themselves suffer from congenital deafness to accepting this possibility in their children. The situation with regard to screening for hip dysplasia is still unresolved.

Adolescence

Although a number of bodies, such as the US Preventive Services Task Force, have suggested several conditions which might be screened for in adolescents, we do not consider that there is adequate evidence for introducing screening services in this age group, with the sole exception of screening for chlamydia.

Adolescence is a time during which there is an opportunity to promote education to prevent smoking, to encourage physical activity and appropriate healthy nutrition, to avoid substance misuse, to promote personal safety and to educate adolescents in the concepts of sexual health and the consequences of unsafe practices. Services need to be easily accessible and friendly, and to provide understandable advice and support. Dental health must be promoted as well as appropriate immunisation. There is a relatively high rate of suicide in this age group, particularly in males. Unfortunately, there are no adequate methods of screening to identify those at highest risk. We consider that easy access to caring, non-judgemental help agencies, along the lines of the Sandyford Initiative discussed in Chapter 5, is crucial here, as is education aimed at increasing self-esteem, rather than the development of population screening with inadequate methods and variable follow-up.

With regard to chlamydia screening, the NSC's position is that a programme of opportunistic screening is being established that will target young people of both sexes under the age of 25 years who access the sexual health services. The phased implementation of the National Chlamydia Screening Programme began in 2002 after successful pilot studies in Portsmouth and Wirral. A total of 26 local chlamydia screening programmes have already been implemented in two phases across England, and a third phase was launched in the autumn of 2004. The objective is to achieve national coverage by 2008 in a way that will avoid unmanaged growth.

Adults

As we stated in Chapter 6, screening in adults is potentially big business as people at this stage of life are increasingly being made aware of potential health problems by the media and private healthcare organisations and are led to believe, often spuriously, that diagnosis by screening will be of benefit.

Despite these pressures, there are only five conditions that, in our view, merit population screening at this stage of life. The national programmes for breast and cervical cancer are well established and should continue, subject to continuing review by the National Screening Committee. Programmes for colorectal cancer in adults aged between 50 and 74 years and for abdominal aortic aneurysm in men aged 65 years or over are on the agenda and awaiting specific recommendations from the NSC. A national programme of screening for diabetic retinopathy for all known diabetics over the age of 12 years is being planned and implemented.

We welcome the measured approach to implementation being adopted by the NSC in relation to the last three programmes. This should help to ensure that adequate facilities and resources are in place for screening to be implemented effectively.

Risk factors for heart disease and stroke – notably, raised blood pressure and cholesterol levels and smoking – should be the subject of case finding and surveillance in primary care, and are part of the Diabetic, Heart Disease and Stroke Prevention Project that is currently being piloted.

Old age

Screening in the elderly for conditions such as cancer or high blood pressure is no different from screening in middle age. Chapter 7 outlines the conditions and tests that we consider to be useful and important. This age group has a much higher rate of use of general practitioner services, so is ideally suited for opportunistic screening or case finding.

The conditions which are most neglected and which cause much concern to the elderly are hearing and visual defects. Any opportunity to detect these during a routine visit should be taken. Other physical conditions, such as asymptomatic bacteriuria, diabetes, anaemia, atrial fibrillation and thyroid dysfunction, should also always be considered by the GP and appropriately investigated. Foot problems and incontinence (particularly in elderly women) may cause much distress and are often 'hidden' by the elderly person, so should be sought in consultations. With computerised records now being used in most general practices it is relatively easy to 'flag' the patient records to remind the nurse or general practitioner to ask the relevant questions at periodic intervals, and to record any findings which may need action at a later date or act as an aide-memoire for increased surveillance.

There is no good evidence for an appropriate screening tool for mental problems such as dementia or depression, which are common among the elderly. However, GPs should be aware of the possibility of these conditions and must look out for them. Simple questions about diet and social isolation may reveal easily remediable problems and help to improve quality of life.

Thus case finding and simple tests for vision, hearing and foot problems and alleviation of social isolation are in our view likely to be far more effective in improving the quality of life and maintaining the dignity of the elderly than the use of myriad screening tests.

Screening practices in Europe

We have included a short chapter on screening practices in six European countries. This can only be a brief overview. The countries concerned have widely differing systems of healthcare and policies on screening. Despite current criticisms of the UK National Health Service, the structure and performance of screening services in the UK and the rigorous scrutiny to which any proposal for a new programme is subjected could serve as a model for other countries.

Table 9.1 Six recommendations for improvement in screening practice in the UK[7]

Number	Recommendation
1	One senior person in each local health authority to coordinate screening activities
2	Satisfactory population registers with call/recall facilities in every general practice
3	Screening process must be adapted to the needs of the specific population within nationally agreed guidelines
4	Long-established criteria for screening must be observed, including the availability of effective treatment
5	Proper evaluation of existing screening procedures is essential, and screening must be subject to medical audit
6	A body should be established with overall responsibility for screening policy and specific responsibility for identifying screening procedures to be included in routine healthcare programmes and those which should be available only on request and possibly on payment of a charge

Conclusions

Much has improved in the organisation of screening in the UK since our previous book, even if the substance and number of programmes are largely the same. This is not the place to comment on the many changes that have occurred in the organisation of the NHS as a whole in the past 15 years, but it is interesting to look back at our six 1990 recommendations, which are summarised in Table 9.1.

The most significant change during the last 15 years has been the establishment in 1996 of the UK National Screening Committee (NSC), which has overall responsibility for screening policy and for identifying screening procedures that should be provided by the NHS. This Committee, as we have shown, has accepted the long-established criteria for the assessment of appropriate tests, and has been effective in commissioning good-quality research where required and in maintaining continuing surveillance and review of function of existing programmes. The Prostate Cancer Risk Management Programme is an example of work aimed at providing advice and testing to those who request it, rather than introducing a national screening programme for which there is insufficient evidence of benefit.

Through the changes in the structure of the NHS, population registers have been introduced in all general practices, thus facilitating adequate call/recall systems. Screening has also been adapted to the particular needs of differing local populations in various parts of the country, and the NSC has been effective in ensuring checks on the quality of screening services and their evaluation, including medical audit.

This has led to a more coordinated and measured approach to screening, with gradual roll-out of several programmes to ensure effective implementation and to avoid overloading the health service.

All this is welcome, but screening remains far from perfect. There is a need for good research, but funding is difficult to find. Screening research is subsumed under the title of Health Services Research but it is expensive to carry out, large numbers of subjects are needed and it takes a long time to produce results. Precedence in funding tends to be given to studies of greater political significance, such as waiting-list targets, where results can be expected more quickly.

Although there is increasing concern with establishing the strength of evidence before introducing a particular screening test, and more emphasis is placed on possible adverse effects, the dilemma of whether the NHS should provide a specific test, even if it has not met the criteria, has not been satisfactorily resolved. One example here is the demand for PSA testing, which was discussed in more detail in Chapter 6. More attention also needs to be paid to the opportunity costs of screening and to the fact that screening may actually increase health inequalities because of differential access and uptake between the affluent and the more deprived groups in the population.

There is also the possibility that the rhetoric behind the introduction of a screening programme may not match the reality of its implementation in practical terms. This can be illustrated by the experience with regard to the introduction of screening for diabetic retinopathy in Glasgow.[8] This is currently being implemented in Scotland with single-field photography without dilatation. There are problems with high rates of non-attendance and technical failure which were not taken into account in the original costings. Recruitment and retention of Grade 1 screening staff is also proving difficult. Another concern with the camera-screening service is that an excessive number of patients with small defects will be referred, overloading secondary care services which are already under pressure. While working to implement the programme successfully, Wykes considers that a better balance would have been struck had screening been performed by optomotrists based in the community.[8]

In 1990, we stated that 'our overall aim for the next decade must be to ensure that screening is used effectively with good organisation and scientific evaluation so that it proves to be a benefit rather than a bane to the health of the population.' This aim has largely been achieved, but more subtle challenges remain.

The first of these is undoubtedly the growth of private screening and full-body checks and the increase in demand from the public in the mistaken hope that screening will ensure future good health. A recent survey of screening in the consumer magazine *Which?* asked two screening experts to provide a verdict on the information and tests provided by five private full-body screening services.[9] They concluded that information provided about the likely benefits, harms and limitations of the tests was in most cases inadequate or even misleading, and they expressed major misgivings about the value of paying for full-body scans. However, it was of interest that the two laypeople who were interviewed for the survey were enthusiastic about screening, highlighting the gap between professional and public perceptions.

Screening provided by the NHS may not be perfect, but it has been introduced on the basis of sound scientific evidence, is subject to ongoing scrutiny and provides continuity of care and follow-up.

Secondly, we must continue to work on the information provided by the NHS screening services about the various programmes and tests to make it understandable and accurate, and to train or retrain those providing it in how to communicate clearly and without bias. It is essential that those who are invited to participate in screening are enabled to make an informed choice with full awareness of all the implications. This will not be easy – particularly, for example, in long-established programmes such as cervical cancer screening, where in some places it is still perceived that women should agree to screening when invited.

It must also be acknowledged that some of the tests involved are extremely unpleasant. Faecal occult blood testing for colorectal cancer is relatively simple and non-invasive (although not appealing). However, colonoscopy, which is the next step after a positive result, most certainly is not.

Thirdly, there is still great variability in the take-up of screening between different parts of the country and different socio-economic groups. It is worrying that the more affluent members of the population who are generally at lower risk are more likely to accept invitations for screening, whereas those in the more deprived sectors who are at higher risk are less likely to do so. Strategies for improving equity of access must be devised and implemented.

Finally, there is a major task involved in educating and informing the media and the public about what screening can and cannot do. Screening is not and never can be a universal remedy but, if used selectively and on the basis of sound research evidence, it can continue to be a good use of resources. Provided that it remains open to constant review and critical evaluation and is capable of change in the light of new evidence, screening will remain a powerful tool in the fight against disease and its impact for the foreseeable future.

References

1 Raffle AE (2004) Cervical screening (editorial). *BMJ.* **328**: 1272–3.
2 Vineis P, Schulte P and McMichael AJ (2001) Misconceptions about the use of genetic tests in populations. *Lancet.* **357**: 709–12.
3 Fokstre S, Myning J, Meredith L, Ravine D and Harper PS (2001) Eight years' experience of direct molecular testing for myotonic dystrophy in Wales. *J Med Genet.* **38**: E42.
4 Harper PS, Linn C and Crawford D (2000) Ten years of presymptomatic testing for Huntington's disease: the experience of the UK Huntington's Disease Prediction Consortium. *J Med Genet.* **37**: 567–71.
5 Holtzman NA (1996) Medical and ethical issues in genetic screening – an academic view. *Environ Health Perspect.* **104 (Suppl. 5)**: 987–90.
6 Barratt A, Trevena L, Davey HM and McCaffery K (2004) Use of decision aids to support informed choices about screening. *BMJ.* **329**: 507–10.
7 Holland WW and Stewart S (1990) *Screening in Health Care: benefit or bane?* The Nuffield Provincial Hospitals Trust, London.
8 Wykes WN (2004) Personal communication.
9 Which? Consumer Survey (2004) Health screening. *Which? Magazine*, 12 August.

Recommendations for screening by life-cycle stage

Antenatal

Routine

Asymptomatic bacteriuria	Urine test	Early in pregnancy
Risk factors for pre-eclampsia		Early in pregnancy
Anaemia		
Blood group and RhD status		
Hepatitis B	Blood test	Early in pregnancy with effective follow-up for any abnormalities identified
HIV		
Rubella immunity		
Syphilis		
Fetal anomalies		
Anencephaly	Ultrasound and blood test if indicated	Between 18 and 20 weeks with effective follow-up
Spina bifida		
Chromosome abnormalities	Quadruple serum tests and ultrasound	Second trimester with effective follow-up
Down's syndrome		

High risk only

Thalassaemia/sickle-cell disease

Tay–Sachs' disease

Under research review

Duchenne muscular dystrophy

Chlamydia

Gestational diabetes

Fragile X syndrome

Hepatitis C

Genital herpes

HTLV1

Streptococcus B

Neonatal

Routine

Bloodspot for

Phenylketonuria	
Congenital hypothyroidism	
Cystic fibrosis	Must be properly evaluated
Sickle-cell disease	In process of introduction for all newborns

Physical examination

Congenital heart disease	Training programme in physical
Congenital cataract	examination being developed
Cryptorchidism	
Congenital dislocation of the hip/ developmental dysplasia of the hip	Use of ultrasound examination as primary screening test to be evaluated
Other congenital malformations	

Other tests

Hearing impairment	Implementation ongoing

Under research review

Biotinidase deficiency	NSC to keep under review
Congenital adrenal hyperplasia	NSC to keep under review
Duchenne muscular dystrophy	NSC to keep under review

Childhood

Hearing impairment	Follow-up on neonatal programme where indicated
	School-entry 'sweep' test to continue for the time being
	Case finding to identify late-onset or progressive impairment
	Investigation of any children with educational or behavioural problems
Amblyopia and impaired vision	Orthoptist screening in 4- to 5-year-olds as per NSC policy
	Attention to be paid to children who miss this test for any reason
Dental disease	School dental screening mandatory, and should continue but be kept under research review
	Early contact with dentists to be encouraged
	Problems include shortage of NHS dentists and lack of parental compliance, especially among the more deprived
Congenital dislocation of the hip/ developmental dysplasia of the hip	Children identified by neonatal screening to be reviewed
	Parental observations and concerns to be investigated
Deprived, disadvantaged or socially isolated children	Need to identify such children and instigate screening/case finding where relevant

Adolescence

| Chlamydia | Phased implementation of opportunistic screening of those aged 25 years or under who access sexual health services |

Adults

Breast cancer	National programme should be continued but kept under close review, with emphasis on quality control, staff training and good information
Cervical cancer	National programme should be continued, with review of alternative types of tests and of age range of those eligible and frequency of screening. Good information to be a priority
Colorectal cancer	National screening programme by faecal occult blood testing for adults aged 50–74 years would be of benefit. Await specific recommendations of NSC before implementation
Abdominal aortic aneurysm	Ultrasound screening of men aged 65 years or over seems a reasonable proposition provided the necessary resources are in place. Await specific recommendations of NSC before implementation
Diabetic retinopathy	National programme of screening for all diabetics over 12 years of age is being planned and implemented. It is essential to be quite clear about how, when and where screening should happen in order to ensure effective implementation

Risk factors for CHD/ stroke
  Blood pressure
  Cholesterol
  Smoking cessation
  Weight
	Surveillance/case-finding approach in general practice

Elderly

Physical assessment	Mental assessment	Social assessment
Hypertension	Depression	Falls
Early heart failure	Alcohol use	Under-nutrition
Hearing loss		Isolation
Vision loss		
Incontinence		
Lack of physical activity		
Foot problems		
Review of medication		

Index

Page numbers in *italics* refer to tables or figures